THE PCOS FIX

The Complete Guide to Get Rid of Polycystic Ovary Syndrome Naturally, Balance Your Hormones, and Boost Your Fertility

By Maggie Glisson

© **Copyright 2019 by Maggie Glisson - All rights reserved.**

The content contained within this book may not be reproduced, duplicated or transmitted without direct written permission from the author or the publisher.

Under no circumstances will any blame or legal responsibility be held against the publisher, or author, for any damages, reparation, or monetary loss due to the information contained within this book. Either directly or indirectly. You are responsible for your own choices, actions, and results.

Legal Notice:

This book is copyright protected. This book is only for personal use. You cannot amend, distribute, sell, use, quote or paraphrase any part, or the content within this book, without the consent of the author or publisher.

Disclaimer Notice:

Please note the information contained within this document is for educational and entertainment purposes only. All effort has been executed to present accurate, up to date, and reliable, complete information. No warranties of any kind are declared or implied. Readers acknowledge that the author is not engaging in the rendering of legal, financial, medical or professional advice. The content within this book has been derived from various sources. Please consult a licensed professional before attempting any techniques outlined in this book.

By reading this document, the reader agrees that under no circumstances is the author responsible for any losses, direct or indirect, which are incurred as a result of the use of the information contained within this document, including, but not limited to, — errors, omissions, or inaccuracies.

TABLE OF CONTENTS

Introduction 1

Chapter One: My Story 5

Chapter Two: What You Need to Know about PCOS 11

Chapter Three: The Causal Factors of PCOS 18

Chapter Four: The Most Common Symptoms Associated with PCOS, and What You Can Do About Them 25

Chapter Five: Tips to Overcome Stress, Depression, and Low Self-Esteem 34

Chapter Six: Your Fertility 50

Chapter Seven: Your Food Is Your Medicine 59

Chapter Eight: Exercise Is Non-Negotiable 91

Chapter Nine: Quality Sleep Is the Key - Your New Night-time & Morning Routines 98

Chapter Ten: Some Extra Tips and Advice 106

Final Words 115

INTRODUCTION

Let me start by saying that I have been where you are right now. I know how it feels to be searching desperately for a solution, how confusing it can be to dig through articles and research papers to try and understand what you are going through and what you can do to heal. One of the reasons I created this book is to help you navigate your way through the advice and begin overcoming PCOS. Maybe you have picked up this book because your partner or friend has been recently diagnosed with PCOS, and you're looking for helpful information for them. In any case, welcome, and rest assured you will find the information you need in these chapters.

My name is Maggie Glisson. A few years ago, I was diagnosed with polycystic ovary syndrome, or PCOS. At the time, the diagnosis devastated and panicked me. I didn't know where to turn, or who to speak to about my condition. Although I had some awareness of what PCOS was, I did not know anyone who had gone through it. I felt that I was alone facing this struggle.

I would like to reassure you: you are not alone. In fact, PCOS affects 1 in 10 women of childbearing age. You will probably have been told that PCOS is not curable. Again, let me reassure you: PCOS is a treatable condition. There may not be a cure, but the strategies in this book will help alleviate your symptoms, rebalance your hormones, and improve your chances of a happy, healthy pregnancy. A PCOS diagnosis is not the end. It is the beginning.

I know, I didn't believe it either when I was first told. But even modern medicine is catching up and realizing that reproductive health is dependent not just on general health, but also mindset, and environment. In order to see significant results, we need a holistic approach to this condition. This means an approach that includes diet, lifestyle, and mindset. Of course, after a PCOS diagnosis it is tempting to reach for the pharmaceuticals, but in truth they will only take you so far. On the other hand, changing your daily habits in a sustainable way will help you overcome PCOS and stop the symptoms from ruling your life.

I wrote this book as a "gateway drug" to the online and offline PCOS community. When I was first diagnosed, it was an uphill struggle to source reliable and supportive information from my doctor. So I searched online and found the answers. I soon recognized that my situation was indicative of a much broader societal problem. The symptoms and implications of PCOS are wide-ranging, regularly undiagnosed, and often disastrous to a whole array of areas, including personal relationships, self-development, and mental wellbeing. The good news is that there is a beautiful community of women who have gone through this or are going through this, and a huge body of information and support in the form of blogs, videos, articles, books and Facebook groups.

My aim here is not to disregard or condense all of that available information. Instead, it is to give you a strong foundation of understanding and knowledge about what you are currently going through, and practical steps to banish PCOS from your life. This is just the first step to a vibrant, healthy, happy tomorrow.

I hope this book will also give you the courage to discuss this subject more freely in your personal life. PCOS can affect as many as 26% of women, so the chances that other amazing women in your life are going through this as well are high. That is why this movement is so important, that is why sharing real, helpful information is so important. And that is why I am so proud and honored to help you take this first step on the road to wellness.

It is so important for us to come together to share our stories and help other women with PCOS. Reading about how something as simple as a blog post or a YouTube video has unlocked the magic key to transforming a PCOS sufferer's life is what gave me the motivation to compile this book.

In the next few chapters, you'll discover:

- Life-changing information about how your sleep, diet, and even your thoughts are contributing to your symptoms
- How PCOS develops, and how to deal with your diagnosis

- The everyday lifestyle habits that cause hormone imbalances and PCOS
- The forgotten link between stress, mindset, and PCOS
- Simple strategies you can begin implementing right now that will deliver real results
- How to easily transform your diet to banish PCOS symptoms and improve your fertility
- Exercise hacks that will get you excited about working out (and there's no need to go to the gym!)
- How to engage with the wider PCOS community and be an inspiration for other women
- How to gain the courage to change your life, start a family, and share your story

If you're ready to kick PCOS out of your life, then reading this book is the first part of that journey.

Let's get started!

Maggie

CHAPTER ONE:

MY STORY

I hope you don't mind if I begin by sharing my journey. It isn't an extraordinary story, I know many women who have gone through the same thing. It's probably just like your story. There is nothing distinctive about me in the same way that there is nothing distinctive about any of us in terms of suffering from PCOS.

Doctors don't fully understand what causes PCOS, but in some ways that does not actually matter. What matters is how we treat it, grow from it, and overcome it; how we learn to identify and acknowledge the symptoms, and how we can educate ourselves and change our behavior to minimize their effects. And that is the reason why I am sharing this with you: to show that it is possible for a normal, everyday woman like me or you, or any of us, to learn to accept, to change, and to eradicate the effects of PCOS in our everyday lives.

My story started just over five years ago. I was in my early thirties, and my partner and I had been trying to get pregnant for around a year. We were not particularly worried at that point; I had only stopped taking the contraceptive pill about a year before that, and we were aware that it could take around a year for my fertility to get back to normal. So the first trip to the doctor to discuss our progress was not particularly worrying. I expected it to be an informal chat about my health ending with a green light to continue our baby-making efforts, safe in the knowledge that time was all that was needed to solve this problem.

Instead, it ended up being an in-depth fact-finding mission that involved uncomfortable questions about my health—areas that I knew had been an issue but in no way thought were related to my chances of getting pregnant. But as he asked question after question, and as I reflected on my general, mental, and physical health, a cold feeling crept over my entire body to the point that when he finished speaking, I was sure I hadn't heard a word he'd said for the last twenty minutes. It was as if it all finally made sense, and I had known all along that there must be some connection between all these facets of my life.

As a teenager, it felt like my life was governed by two things: my weight and my emotions. With a diet sky-high in sugar and processed food and with years to go before the average person knew about the impact these foods would have, I was completely ignorant about the effects my lifestyle choices were having on my long-term health. My mood swings and tendency to burst into tears at a moment's notice were labelled as a normal part of puberty. This theory was backed up by the fact that so many of my girlfriends seemed to be going through similar experiences. We were assured by parents, teachers, and each other that this was all just part of growing up, and as soon as we were older, our bodies would normalize and our emotions would even out.

Fast forward to my mid-twenties, where my body had normalized for sure. My new normal was an extra 15-25 pounds that I carried mostly around my stomach. It became so normal I stopped noticing. Every few years, I would creep up a dress size. I would jump from one fad diet to another with no results other than an extra few pounds. This was due in part to the fact that I never stuck to one dietary plan for long, and that whenever I tried to cut down on sugary treats or bread, I would be so miserable that I would quickly pick it back up again.

Again, most of my girlfriends had the same issues. This was back in the days when the internet had just cemented itself as a part of our daily routines, and social media was starting to grow popular. So, I could see that not only were some of the women in my family and social circle prone to weight gain but other women as well! This pattern only added to my confidence that there was nothing wrong with me in particular—weight gain, and what seemed like complete immunity to the effects of exercise were just normal parts of being in your twenties. Plus, by that point, I had already met my husband-to-be, and we were happy. So why worry so much about my weight if there was nothing I could do to change it?

The emotional symptoms were a bit harder to explain away. I had progressed out of the teenage phase of bursting into tears at the drop of a hat, but that had been replaced with a slow-growing, ever-present, and sometimes overwhelming feeling of unhappiness and discontent. It grew so steadily during my early twenties that I almost didn't notice it. But by the time I was approaching my thirties, getting married, and considering starting a family, it had taken over so much of my thought process and mental health that I had already reached out to medical professionals for help.

As a woman in her late twenties, I was now refusing to hear that my problems were normal or that I would grow out of them. My thirties were approaching. Surely my time for growing out of things was long behind me! Some of the strategies I tried worked temporarily, some didn't work at all, and others I refused to even try. Again, as with the weight, after a while I assumed that this was just the way I was. And hey, every couple argued, and there were times when I was upset over things that could be considered legitimate concerns. No way could this all be connected to any physical problem. This was just part of life.

Now into my early thirties, imagine my moment of absolute clarity in that doctor's office when my answers to all of his questions around my health were that it was *"Just the way I was."* The weight; the depression; the emotional overreaction; the acne; the debilitating pain during my period; the irregular and sometimes absent periods; the irrational fights with my husband. These things were not just me being me—these were symptoms. These were symptoms of PCOS that I had actually been trying to normalize from when I was 13 years old.

Getting a medical diagnosis can feel like you have the proverbial weight taken off your shoulders. But realizing that this diagnosis could now spell infertility was like having that weight, and then some, replaced. Okay, this was my life now. This was us starting the journey of looking at other medical options in order to get pregnant. This was our time to start using the words in vitro fertilization, surrogacy, or even adoption.

Or was it?

Over the years, I had researched natural treatments for my depressive episodes and general mental health. In the process, I had become increasingly aware of holistic approaches for a wide range of female health conditions. I started to think about the information I might find if I looked into possible treatments for PCOS. Was there a chance that maybe, just maybe, I would be able to heal, and possibly even have a family naturally?

And so I began my journey into the online world of PCOS information and support. It is a journey that I am still on to this very day, although my reasons for continuing this journey have changed. You see, I've already received my miracle. I have a healthy, happy baby who was conceived naturally and delivered with no complications. For many women, their PCOS journey would have ended there. But for me, it was not just about achieving that goal, although I can't even tell you how much joy and happiness our son has brought in to our lives. For me, it was also about getting my life back: enjoying great health, learning to love myself, and improving my personal relationships. That part of my journey surprised me the most.

That is why I have made it my mission to share my knowledge and experience with other women like you. That is why I now feel confident and empowered to share my story. If becoming pregnant is your goal, then this book can help with that. But there is more to PCOS than fertility problems, and I want to raise awareness of how recognizing, managing, and overcoming the symptoms of PCOS will radically transform almost every area of your life.

Thank you for taking the time to read my story. Now, let's dive in and really explore what we are dealing with when we talk about PCOS.

CHAPTER TWO:

WHAT YOU NEED TO KNOW ABOUT PCOS

Great! Let's get started! First of all, I think it is important for us to look at what PCOS is and how it affects your body. I am also aware that some women reading this book are undiagnosed (you're not alone, some studies show that up to 70% of PCOS sufferers don't know they have it). If so, you might be looking for clues as to whether PCOS might be affecting you before going to a medical professional. We will also take some time to delve into the symptoms and how to spot it early.

Before we start with what PCOS is, I think it is important to consider what it most definitely is NOT. Most importantly, it is *not* your fault. In the following pages you might read warning signs and obvious manifestations of PCOS that ring so true that you might wonder why you never noticed it earlier. You'll also learn about the causes and might feel that you have done this to yourself. Thinking in this manner can lead to a negative spiral of self-doubt and blame. I know that was my first thought. *How could I not have known sooner?* But actually, it is so common for symptoms to go unrecognized that not noticing or suspecting any abnormalities is the norm. When I learned about the changes that have the biggest positive impact on PCOS symptoms, such as regular exercise, stress-busting meditations, a plant-based diet, I felt depressed because I realized that I had many of the answers all along, but not the motivation. However, when I started putting these strategies into practice and experiencing the physical and emotional benefits, this no longer mattered. Right now, it doesn't matter how you arrived here. This is not a time to feel guilty or to blame yourself. All that matters is that you're here, with this book in your hand, and you're about to transform your health for the better. No more excuses, it is time to take your health into your hands.

It is certainly not the intention of this book, and never my intention personally, to make anyone feel that they could have done something sooner or that this could have been avoided, and we can all agree that type of thinking is far from helpful. Let us instead agree that your PCOS recovery journey starts here, and everything else that we believed, practiced, or avoided in the past was actually a necessary part of the journey because it brought us here, to this moment of awareness, acceptance, and the start of immense positive change.

For such an important and far-reaching condition, it is surprising just how common PCOS is. When you first got diagnosed, you might not have even heard of PCOS before, and you might have assumed it was a rare and uncommon condition. You might be surprised to learn that a lot of women in your social circle and even your family have lived with this syndrome and just never talked about it. Thankfully we now live in a time where we can find support circles and communities online. Once you start looking in these areas, you will be amazed at just how many women PCOS affects, and until recently, how little awareness there was about managing PCOS through lifestyle, diet, and exercise.

Okay. Now we have that out of the way, let's dive into what PCOS really is, how it is diagnosed, why it is commonly misdiagnosed and underdiagnosed, and the many different forms that it takes. This is the perfect time to grab a hot drink, get comfortable, and begin.

What Is PCOS?

Let's start with the term itself: **P**oly-**C**ystic **O**vary **S**yndrome. The term "poly" means "many", so PCOS refers to the presence of many cysts growing in the ovaries. But what are these cysts, and how else does PCOS manifest?

Ovaries are the reproductive organs that produce the sex hormones estrogen and progesterone, which regulate the menstrual cycle. They also produce a small amount of androgen hormones (male hormones like testosterone).

Every month, the ovaries ovulate: they release an egg, ready to be fertilized by sperm. This process of releasing an egg is controlled by follicle-stimulating hormone (FSH) and luteinizing hormone (LH). FSH stimulates the ovary to produce a follicle (a sac containing an immature egg), while LH stimulates the ovary to release the egg once it is mature.

The cysts in the ovaries are actually follicles. The eggs do no achieve maturity and therefore do not trigger ovulation. This lack of ovulation then has a knock-on effect: it lowers the levels of estrogen, progesterone, follicle-stimulating hormone and luteinizing hormone, while increasing the level of androgen hormones.

This increase in androgen hormones disrupts the menstrual cycle, which is why women with PCOS tend to have fewer or irregular periods (one of the most obvious signs that something is wrong with your cycle and your fertility), while also increasing the likelihood of other symptoms such as facial hair and acne.

PCOS is first and foremost a hormonal issue. Hormones are messengers - they tell your body to do certain things. If they are out of balance, this has far reaching consequences on your health - not just your reproductive health, but your overall wellbeing. It can be a debilitating condition, and it manifests in various ways. Let's take a closer look at the symptoms.

What Are the Symptoms?

PCOS is a "syndrome," or group of symptoms that affects the ovaries and ovulation. Its three main features are:

- Cysts in the ovaries
- High levels of male hormones
- Irregular or skipped periods

These features come with a number of other physical and mental manifestations due to imbalanced hormones:

- Heavy bleeding (due to the lining of the uterus building up over a longer period of time and leading to heavier periods)
- Acne (androgens make skin oilier and more prone to breakouts)
- Hirsutism (excess hair growing on face, back, chest, stomach)
- Hair loss (male pattern baldness)
- Excess weight (around 80% of women with PCOS are overweight)
- Darkening of skin (PCOS can cause dark patches of skin to appear, particularly around creases such as the neck, breasts and groin)
- Depression and anxiety (PCOS symptoms such as acne and weight gain increase the likelihood of mood disorders)
- Difficulty conceiving (trying for 12 months unsuccessfully)

Looking at this list, it's easy to see how PCOS can impact your self-confidence. Low self-esteem negatively impacts all areas of your life. Unfortunately, this becomes a bit of a negative downward spiral. The lower you feel, the more likely you are to partake in behaviors that make the condition worse. For example, you might reach for comfort foods, which increase weight gain and insulin sensitivity, and disrupt your hormones. We will look at the causes of PCOS in more detail in the next chapter. But before we do, I'd like to reassure you that rebalancing your hormones, losing weight, clearing up your skin, improving your fertility and banishing depression are all possible with the right lifestyle strategies and a few dietary changes.

Living with PCOS can be unbearable. I experienced a number of these symptoms in varying stages and to varying degrees, and, for me, the emotional symptoms were the worst. Before I understood that they were due to an actual medical condition, I believed my issues were untreatable and something that I and those closest to me would just have to learn to live with. My first miracle was realizing that there was a name for everything that was happening to me, and the second miracle was realizing that it could be healed with choices I made every single day. There's hope, and that's what this book is about.

How Is PCOS Diagnosed?

We have become so used to having irregular periods and mood-swings that most of us don't even consider we might have PCOS, even though the symptoms manifest in our everyday lives. This is one of the major reasons why most PCOS sufferers are undiagnosed. It often isn't until a woman wants to conceive that she will see a doctor and discover there are problems.

Diagnosing PCOS is relatively straightforward, but has to be carried out by a medical professional. Self-diagnosing is not reliable. Although of course, self-awareness helps. If you are unsure whether you have PCOS or not, be mindful of the changes in your body. Have you noticed any of the symptoms listed above? A doctor will carry out one of three tests to check whether you have PCOS:

- Blood tests - these will check for levels of male hormones. High levels of androgens will indicate PCOS.
- Ultrasound - this will detect any cysts or problems with your ovaries.
- Pelvic exam - the doctor will check for growths in your ovaries and uterus.

For younger women, or women who have never been sexually active, it is possible to identify PCOS with only an ultrasound, so don't worry about having to endure invasive procedures. The combination of all three diagnostic tests is the perfect trifecta of proof, but a doctor will also be able to provide a clear diagnosis of PCOS using only one or two of these methods.

In this chapter, we have looked at some of the important points you need to know about PCOS. In the next chapters, we will go into each of these areas in much more detail, both to explain what is going on, and give you easy-to-implement tips and strategies to help you redress those symptoms. There is no magic cure for PCOS. It's about taking an honest look at how you live your life right now, and being ready to make changes to your habits and routines. Don't worry if you're feeling overwhelmed - just take it one step at a time. Before you know it, you'll be feeling healthier than ever.

CHAPTER THREE:

THE CAUSAL FACTORS OF PCOS

There is no single cause for PCOS. Instead, there are several factors that most experts agree contribute significantly to the presence, development, and severity of PCOS and its symptoms. These three factors are genetics, insulin resistance, and inflammation. Now, you might think that not much can be done about these things, so allow me to reassure you. Your health is firmly in your hands. You have the power to improve your wellbeing with the right diet and lifestyle.

When I first started learning about PCOS, it took me on a journey of discovery unlike anything I had experienced before. I quickly became obsessed with understanding how my body worked and the importance of food, movement and stress. Just remember as you read this chapter that we will only spend a short time looking at the things we have no control over before switching to the things that we do have control over.

As you begin to implement the changes suggested in this and the following chapters, you will notice a gradual improvement in your PCOS symptoms, particularly when it comes to skin, mood, and excess weight. Let's take a look at each of these three factors in turn.

Genetics

Many genes are responsible for the occurrence of PCOS, but the exact mechanism by which this happens is still unclear. Some studies show that PCOS runs in families, so if you have a family history of the condition, you are more likely to experience it yourself. However, this is not a doom and gloom scenario. We know that genes are only a tiny part of the issue. There's a saying in the scientific community: Genes load the gun, lifestyle pulls the trigger. What this means is that while you might have certain genes that pre-dispose you to hormone imbalances, your lifestyle can turn those genes on or off. In other words: your genes don't control your health, you do.

For example, you might have the gene that increases your likelihood of insulin resistance (the second major factor in PCOS, which we'll look at next), while your friend doesn't. Having that gene doesn't automatically mean your insulin levels will be too high. You can mitigate that possibility by ensuring you eat foods that do not lead to a spike in insulin. In the same token, even if you don't have that gene, a diet packed with processed foods and high-sugar foods will result in insulin resistance.

This is good news for you. Even if a close family member has had PCOS, this doesn't necessarily mean you can't overcome it. And when you do, you will be able to share these strategies and help your loved ones improve their health as well.

Insulin Resistance

To understand how insulin resistance impacts your hormones, we first need to look at the role insulin plays in the body.

Insulin is a hormone that is secreted by your pancreas and is involved in energy production and storage.

When you eat carbohydrates, your digestive system converts them into glucose, which is your cells' preferred form of fuel. This glucose is dumped into the bloodstream, ready to be used for energy. The pancreas then releases insulin. Insulin tells your cells to open up and absorb the glucose. If the carbohydrates you eat are healthy (for example complex carbohydrates that have a good ratio of starch and fiber), then only a little insulin is needed. However, when you eat a lot of sugar (and unfortunately our modern diets are packed with the stuff), your pancreas has to pump out more and more insulin to help get all that glucose out of the bloodstream. Your body can cope with that happening every so often, but if there is regularly too much sugar in the diet, your cells stop responding to insulin - they become resistant to insulin's signaling. This is known as insulin resistance, and it is a precursor for Type 2 diabetes, which is why many women with PCOS are either diabetic or at risk of becoming diabetic.

Insulin also happens to be the fat storing hormone, and that is why many women with PCOS also struggle with excess weight. When there is too much glucose in the blood, insulin signals to the body to store it as adipose tissue (fat cells). This is how sugar, which ironically is fat-free, makes us fat. And as we saw, excess weight is one of the symptoms associated with PCOS.

Interestingly, insulin resistance also creates imbalances of other hormones, for example testosterone. While testosterone is technically a male hormone, it is also present, in small amount, in women, and plays a role in healthy muscle mass, circulatory system, and libido. But balance is key. Increased levels of testosterone can lead to problems such as amenorrhea (lack of periods), acne, and facial hair. Other factors can contribute to higher levels of testosterone, for example high levels of stress.

The good news is that even if you are insulin resistant, you can turn things around with your next meal. And as you get your insulin levels under control, your weight will normalize, and your hormone levels will become more balanced.

What Causes Insulin Resistance?

Very simply: too much sugar. And you might be surprised where sugar lurks. In salad dressings, in ready meals, even in some vitamins! You can rest assured that if you eat processed foods, you're eating more sugar than is ideal for health.

According to health authorities, women should eat no more than 25 grams of added sugar a day (around 6 teaspoons).

Added sugar refers to sugar added to food, rather than sugar that is naturally present in food (for example the naturally present sugars in an apple). But the average consumption of added sugar is closer to 80 grams per day. No wonder we're seeing a global obesity epidemic.

And it's no wonder most people go over. A 12-oz can of regular coke contains 39 grams of sugar, almost double the recommended intake.

In Chapter 7, you'll find a list of healthy alternatives so you can swap high-sugar foods with foods that are lower in sugar and higher in other nutrients that help slow down the release of glucose, thereby redressing insulin resistance and helping you lose weight naturally.

Inflammation

Studies have found that women with PCOS often have high levels of inflammation in their body. Now, what does this mean?

Inflammation is your body's natural way to heal. Think about when you cut yourself, for example while chopping carrots. Your immune system instantly realizes something is wrong, and mobilizes. It sends immune cells (white blood cells and inflammatory cytokines) to the site of injury to fight any infection, surround the area, and begin the healing process. Once the cut has healed, the inflammation goes away. This is known as acute inflammation.

But the inflammation we're talking about here is known as chronic inflammation, and is rather different in so far as it does the opposite of healing. Chronic inflammation happens when the immune system is on constant high alert in response to triggers such as artificial additives or allergens in food, pollution in the air, or chemicals in your toiletries. Scientists consider this type of inflammation as a key contributor to the development of PCOS, because high levels of inflammatory cytokines stimulate the body's production of androgen hormones. Excess weight also contributes to high levels of inflammation, and can therefore exacerbate the hormonal imbalances seen in PCOS. But it doesn't stop there - in fact, this type of inflammation is understood to underpin almost all lifestyle diseases, from heart disease to cancer. It is therefore imperative to get inflammation under control - not just to banish PCOS symptoms and improve your fertility, but also for your future health.

And here again, there is hope. Because three times a day you can choose foods that give your body the nourishment to cool down this inflammation and rebalance your hormones.

What Causes Chronic Inflammation?

Unfortunately, the very way we live contributes to chronic inflammation. We have swapped natural, whole foods for foods that are mixed with artificial ingredients and wrapped in plastic. We breathe air that is heavy with pollution. We are stressed almost 24/7. All of this triggers the immune system into action - and because these triggers are always present, it can never relax. It's a bit like an office worker: it has a job to do and it does it. But what would happen if every day someone dumped a mountain of files on the desk, and did so relentlessly? For the first few weeks, the office worker can cope - it can grab a coffee or two, speed up its output, and carry on. But in time, it becomes exhausted. It begins making mistakes. That's what happens with your immune system. The files being relentlessly dumped on the desk are processed foods, chemicals, pollution, plastics; and the result is chronic inflammation, which opens the door to hormonal imbalances and a host of other problems from autoimmune conditions to cancer.

This is why it is imperative that you reduce the triggers. The good news is that, armed with the right information, you can make better choices about what you put on your plate and what you put in your mind. And, through that, you can banish PCOS symptoms and improve your overall wellbeing.

I hope that this chapter has given you an insight into the main areas thought to cause PCOS and a better understanding of how these issues then affect your symptoms. In the next chapter, we are going to look at these symptoms in much greater detail, and strategies to get rid of them.

CHAPTER FOUR:

THE MOST COMMON SYMPTOMS ASSOCIATED WITH PCOS, AND WHAT YOU CAN DO ABOUT THEM

We've briefly touched on the common symptoms associated with PCOS. In this section, let's look at these more closely, discuss the conventional approaches, and explore some ways you can make yourself more comfortable and begin the healing process.

You may already be familiar with some of the content that will be discussed in this chapter. I had a series of *Aha!* moments as I delved deeper into the common symptoms of PCOS and learned how the condition can present itself in areas not even related to the reproductive system. Being aware of such symptoms and recognizing the effects that they can have in your daily life is an important step to overcoming them. Pharmaceutical options are available, but they come with side effects and fail to address the underlying causes behind PCOS. This makes them at best a temporary solution. My aim with this book is not to replace medical advice, only to give you the information you need to make conscious choices about your health and your body.

Menstrual Cycle

The first area of your life in which physical symptoms of PCOS present themselves is your menstrual cycle. PCOS typically comes with irregular periods, for example every three weeks or every five, or in some cases no periods at all. The first remedy prescribed by doctors to balance this is some form of contraceptive. Unfortunately, while contraceptive pills can regularize periods, they also mask the problem - unbalanced hormones - and many women find that when they stop taking the pill, they struggle to conceive. Contraceptive pills also do nothing to address inflammation or insulin resistance. These are issues that can be remedied through diet, exercise, and proper sleep - and you'll discover the best strategies for all these aspects in the next few chapters.

A menstrual cycle of more than 35 days is a common sign that you have PCOS. Other signs include heavy bleeding for more than seven days, or pain elsewhere in your body when menstruating, such as tender breasts. Women with PCOS can also have a complete absence of menses. As you can see, there are multiple ways in which your menstrual cycle could be giving you signs that something isn't quite right.

A good way to start healing is to monitor your cycle. It's ok if you haven't been doing this, you can begin today. Write down the date and length of your last period in a calendar. You can keep a cycle diary, where you record the dates of your periods and how you feel day by day. This doubles up nicely as a food diary. Keeping track of things - your cycle, the foods you eat, the exercise you do, and how you feel physically and emotionally, helps you to reconnect with your health and discover which strategies and foods make you feel good, and which ones don't. In this way, you can begin to track your progress as you shift your lifestyle to one that balances your hormones.

Weight

Around 80% of women with PCOS are overweight or obese. This means a BMI of over 24 (overweight) or 31 (obese). If you're unsure whether you fall into this category, there are hundreds of free BMI calculators online - simply enter your height and weight. I was overweight, and carried most of my weight around my middle - a term known as apple shaped. This is common. Insulin resistance often goes hand in hand with visceral fat. Visceral fat is a term used to describe fat around your mid-section, and is more dangerous than body fat because it is concentrated around your vital organs.

Weight is not a genetic issue, although many people think that weight issues are beyond their control. I certainly did. It felt as though no matter how much I worked out or the fad diets I went on, my weight crept steadily upwards. I figured this was just the way it was, maybe I was supposed to be bigger. Perhaps you have had the same experience - trying multiple diets and exercise plans only to feel discouraged and put it to slow metabolism or genes.

Excess weight is a symptom of two things: too many poor-quality calories (empty calories from cakes, biscuits, fizzy drinks, processed foods, etc.) and too many toxins (from artificial additives, environmental pollutants and chemicals in toiletries). We saw in the last chapter that a diet high in sugar causes high levels of insulin, which then signals to the body to store excess glucose as fat. The result: weight gain. Adipose tissue (fat tissue) is also the body's repository for the toxins it cannot process or eliminate. The more toxins you come into contact with, the heavier you become.

This is then compounded by PCOS in two ways. Firstly, through hyperandrogenism (when you have an excess of male hormones in your body) which can cause an accumulation of visceral fat. Secondly, through depression, since most of us will comfort eat to sooth the discomfort of PCOS symptoms, thereby making it more likely we will gain more weight.

So it is clear that losing weight has to go beyond simply counting calories or diet pills. Calorie counting ignores the health value to a food (for example, 300 calories from an avocado will have a significantly different impact on your body compared with 300 calories from a bag of sweets). Diet pills do not address the reasons for the excess weight, and they come with a long list of side effects, from digestive trouble to heart palpitations.

Sustainable, healthy weight loss is achieved through a combination of strategies: avoiding processed foods and foods that spike your insulin; favoring foods that keep your blood sugar and your hormones balanced; and using ingredients that help your body detoxify. Exercise is also a vital part of this journey - but don't worry, I hated exercise too. In Chapter 8 I'll show you ways you can trick yourself into falling in love with working out.

Begin keeping a food diary today. It is very easy to underestimate how much we eat, and you might be keeping yourself in the dark about your food habits without even realizing it. Write down what you eat, the time you eat it, and how you feel before and after you eat it. This will give you an honest and accurate picture of your dietary habits right now, and help you identify any food sensitivities as well (food sensitivities can increase chronic inflammation). With that awareness, it will be much easier to transition to foods that support your body. Plus, you'll be able to look back, track your progress, and see how far you've come.

Mood

Another noticeable symptom of PCOS is mood swings. You may well have noticed this, and this also impacts your relationships, particularly your partner. These shifts in mood, whether depression or anxiety, are a result of a complex interplay of factors that include hormonal imbalances, poor gut health, and low self-esteem.

The common medical approach is to prescribe SSRI's (selective serotonin re-uptake inhibitors). These are anti-depressants that work by limiting how the brain re-absorbs serotonin (our very own happy-chemical), resulting in higher levels of serotonin in the brain. While that sounds promising, the truth is that our mood depends on much more than just one neurotransmitter, and it certainly depends on more than just our brain. In truth, these medications are not all that effective. In fact, studies have found that they work no better than a placebo. In other words, it is likely that the belief that they will improve mood is what improves mood, rather than the drugs themselves. Unlike a placebo, however, SSRI's have a long list of undesirable side effects, including, ironically enough, depression and anxiety. What's more, some scientists believe that these anti-depressants make people more vulnerable to future mood disorders by creating a dependency.

It is absolutely possible to reconnect with a happier, calmer state of mind without pharmaceuticals. That journey begins with the belief that you are in control of your thoughts and emotions. No matter what happens in your life, you can choose how you react to it. Yes, it's that old cliché: do you choose to see the glass half full, or half empty? Shifting your perspective to one where you seek out the positive in any situation is the first step towards a happier you. Start now. It certainly sucks to have PCOS, and to struggle through all of the symptoms. But what if this is part of a bigger picture?

What if, because of this problem, you find the information and motivation to radically improve your health? What might happen if you began viewing your PCOS as a gift and something to learn from?

In Chapter 5, I'll share tips to help you step out of sadness and worry any time you choose, and strategies to lift your mood generally. But for now, begin keeping track of your emotions by jotting them down in a diary.

Acne, Hirsutism, Hair Thinning

Adult acne, excess facial, and thinning hair are among the most crippling things that can happen to you when it comes to self-confidence. They are typically difficult to hide, and you might feel like you don't want to leave the house. That's how I felt. Sometimes my skin would be so bad that I stayed indoors for weeks at a time.

Low self-esteem holds us back. You may delay going for that job promotion, avoid social situations, or not pursue relationships because of how you feel about your appearance. It also exacerbates depression and anxiety, or at the very least increases your irritability and mood swings.

There are medical options - for example, the contraceptive pill is often prescribed to help clear up acne and PCOS-related hair issues, but as we saw earlier, this only masks the problem. The best strategy for clearing up your skin and helping your hair to regrow is to follow a healthy diet - Chapter 7 has more information on how to do this, but for now I'd like to share three natural supplements that can help clear your skin and regrow your hair:

- Zinc: A study found that women who supplemented with zinc had reduced alopecia (hair loss) and reduced hirsutism. The dose was 220 milligrams zinc sulfate containing 50 milligrams zinc, for 8 weeks.
- Biotin: A review of studies about biotin found that it significantly improves hair condition by increasing hair growth and stopping hair from shedding. It also helps keep your nails strong. Studies showing biotin improvements for alopecia suggest taking up to 10 milligrams of biotin per day.
- Probiotics: Many studies show a direct link between acne and gut dysbiosis - a condition where bad bacteria in your gut outnumber the good bacteria. Probiotic supplements help to restore gut balance and can reduce acne lesions. Choose a lactobacillus-containing supplement, preferably with other strains of bacteria to provide your gut with a good variety.

NB: some supplements can interact with medications. For example, biotin can interact with some anti-convulsant drugs. It's a good idea to speak to your practitioner beforehand, especially if you are taking pharmaceuticals.

Beyond diet and lifestyle, the biggest change you can make to your appearance is actually invisible: it's a change in how you view yourself. If you can view your PCOS with gratitude at the lessons it can teach, then you can include any physical insecurities into that. Feeling insecure about my looks made

me more compassionate towards other people's struggl
forced me to change what I value. Looks, after all, will fac
What remains is a human being, kindness, wisdom, strength, personality… and love. Who are you? You're not your skin or your hair style, you are so much more, and beautiful no matter what. In the next chapter, we're going to dive into finding love for yourself and how you look, no matter what social pressures there are to look a certain way.

One thing that should be becoming clear is that PCOS cannot be treated by addressing one single thing. For example, you can't just take a pill and magically get better. This goes for pharmaceuticals but it also goes for natural healing strategies. Addressing your diet but not sorting out your lifestyle will only go so far. Taking supplements without changing your eating habits won't deliver real results. Exercising while continuing to eat processed foods will not help you get healthy long term. In order to heal PCOS, you have to take a holistic approach. That means addressing all aspects of your life that can impact your hormones. That means diet, mindset, daily habits, and movement. In the next few chapters, we'll get into each of these elements so that you can begin transforming your health for the better.

CHAPTER FIVE:

TIPS TO OVERCOME STRESS, DEPRESSION, AND LOW SELF-ESTEEM

We can all agree that the physical symptoms of PCOS are pretty hard to cope with. When it comes to the mental impact, well, we all know how quickly self-esteem can plummet, and how destructive anxiety and depression can be. It tarnishes everything, from relationships to future prospects. And this is a vicious cycle, because the lower you feel, the less likely you are to take positive action to tackle PCOS.

Maybe these feelings have been a direct result of your PCOS, or maybe they were an underlying issue before your hormones got involved. Perhaps you've tried pharmaceuticals and these aren't helping. Regardless of why you are feeling low, believe me when I tell you that feeling better is within your grasp. And it doesn't depend on anything other than you.

So, in this section I'm going to take a look at the three main factors in anxiety and depression, and offer you some tips so you can banish those negative feelings and feel happier. This will help you to tackle PCOS head on. Because more respect and love you have for yourself, the easier it will be to implement positive changes.

1. Stress - Depression Amplifier and Inflammation Booster

There is no denying we live in stressful times. Most of us rush from morning to evening - rush to work, rush through paperwork, stuff lunch into our faces while checking emails, eat dinner slumped in front of the TV while browsing our social media feeds. This might sound pretty innocuous. But the fact is that this everyday stress is making us sick.

Stress triggers the body's fight-or-flight response. This is a product of evolution, something that kept us safe from predators, back in cave-dwelling times. Imagine yourself a cave woman, foraging for roots. Out of the corner of your eye, you spot a wild bear. Your body instantly reacts: your blood pressure increases to pump blood to your extremities and your heart rate speeds up to pump more oxygen through your body, so that you have the energy to run away or to defend yourself. After the danger passes, your body returns to normal.

These days the predators have different forms. It's the cliff-hanger finale on that Netflix series, the 50 notifications on your phone, the report you have to hand in tomorrow, that guy that cut you up on the motorway, another news report, an unpaid bill. What that means is that most of us are experiencing low-level stress all the time. This is bad news for your health and hormone levels.

One of the ways stress manifests physically is through increased cortisol levels. In small amounts, cortisol helps you focus and makes you clear headed. A little bit of stress can be beneficial - it can be motivating and push you to challenge yourself. Unfortunately, too much cortisol increases inflammation (and as we've seen, inflammation is a factor in PCOS). In a study examining the link between stress and PCOS, researchers found that women with the condition had significantly higher levels of cortisol than healthy women.

What does this tell us? That stress is playing a part in your PCOS. If you're feeling not your best anyway, stress can compound that and make you feel worse. It can also take you by the hand towards bad dietary habits - take away pizza, ice cream and a couple of glasses of wine is not an uncommon result of a bad day at the office. But all that does is lead you down a downward spiral of low mood, irritability, weight gain, and anxiety, and can ultimately ramp up your PCOS symptoms.

It is clear that reducing stress is key to rebalancing your hormones. Ok, so how can you do that? Most of us never really stop, never fully relax, we're always waiting for the next thing, always worrying about tomorrow. This is partly out of our control - deadlines are set by our bosses, modern living is naturally fast paced and demanding, particularly in cities. But the good news is there are many things you can do to protect yourself from stress and get yourself into a mindset where you are able to remain calm even in challenging situations. These strategies are: meditation and mindfulness, gratitude, and proper sleep.

Meditation and Mindfulness

Meditation and mindfulness practices have enjoyed a surge in popularity in recent years, and for a good reason. Science has confirmed what monks and meditators knew all along: that it can have a dramatically positive impact on both your mental and physical health. And the good news is that you don't need to sit cross legged for hours, chanting in a room filled with incense, unless of course you like that. You can begin feeling the benefits of meditation from day one, even if you don't know how to meditate.

Just sitting in a meditative state for 5-10 minutes each day will give you huge results, and you will start to see the benefits after a relatively short period. When I started teaching myself how to meditate, I used the Sam Harris Waking Up app on my phone. It's very helpful to be guided through the process, and it gives you a great starting block, especially if you are not familiar with meditation. Some free apps available like Calm and Headspace offer guided meditations. During a guided meditation, you will be led to visualize a calming scene or push away the thoughts that pop up in your head.

Many people think that meditation refers to not thinking of anything. This is a mistake, and can lead to frustration because, since the very nature of the mind is to think, attempting to stop thinking is a bit like trying to flatten the ocean with an iron. I see meditation as a process, not of emptying the mind, but of witnessing and acknowledging any thoughts that do come up with love and acceptance, without judgement.

Incorporating mindfulness into meditation really helps. We live mostly in our minds, and our minds keep up a constant chatter about all manner of things, some of them rather unhelpful, almost all of it unconscious. We might ruminate on the argument we had with our partner, or the number on the scales this morning, or we might be stuck in the story we tell ourselves about our lives - that nobody can be depended on, that we're alone, that life is hard. The result is that we are disconnected from the present.

Mindfulness is the practice of being fully with whatever it is you're doing. For example, if you're walking, then just walk. Focus on the sensation of your foot on the floor, the way your body is moving, your breathing, how the air smells. Or, if you're preparing vegetables, you allow yourself to be completely present in that action. Not peeling carrots while worrying about tomorrow's to-do list, but instead gently focusing on the carrot and the action of peeling. You'll be surprised how much calmer you feel when you allow yourself some time away from the habitual chatter of your thoughts.

Incorporating a daily meditation and mindfulness routine in your life will help reduce your stress levels. Lower stress levels mean lower levels of cortisol and therefore helps reduce inflammation. Better still, these practices will help you to lift yourself out of depression and anxiety.

Begin with 5 minutes of meditation twice a day. My recommendation would be to meditate in the morning and before going to bed, this way you begin your day centered and calm, and prepare yourself for a restful night's sleep (another key ingredient in your fight against PCOS). You can either use a meditation app or a guided meditation on YouTube. If you prefer silence, simply sit and gently place your attention on your breath. As you notice any thoughts come up, witness them as though they are characters arriving on a stage. Acknowledge them as simply passing thoughts and let them go (I found it helpful to visualize them exiting the stage).

When it comes to mindfulness, you can practice this at any time of day, no matter where you are or what you're doing. Stuck in traffic? Waiting in a queue? House chores to do? Enormous pile of paperwork to get through? Be with it. Observe your surroundings, feel the sensations in your body, observe the thoughts that come up from a space of loving awareness. You'll be surprised how difficult it is to stay in a frustrated mental space when you practice mindfulness.

As you begin any new practice, keep track of your progress in a journal. How do you feel when you meditate, how has your mood evolved, how are your relationships improving? These moments of stillness can bring you a sense of calm, as well as inspiration and clarity. You really have nothing to lose and everything to gain by adding meditation and mindfulness to your day.

Gratitude

I find that I can't talk about meditation and mindfulness without giving a special mention to gratitude. If anything has the power to instantly shift your mood, it's this.

It's funny that, at a time when many of us live in relative abundance and comfort, we are more dissatisfied and depressed than ever. There are several reasons for this. One is the fact we live in a society that values material wealth above all else, and where we are constantly reminded of the things we ought to have in our lives (a new sofa, a faster car, a slimmer figure…). This leads to a sense of discontentment and unease, and contributes to that background stress we all experience.

The antidote is gratitude.

There is no special way to practice gratitude. You can do it anytime, anywhere, and anyhow. You can practice it by looking someone in the eye when you say thank you. You can hit the snooze button on your alarm clock and use those first five minutes to contemplate what you are grateful for in that moment. You can make mental gratitude lists as you go about your day. You might combine mindfulness with gratitude - for example spending time in a field full of flowers and feeling grateful to Mother Nature for making the world so breathtakingly beautiful, or for the warm rays of sunshine on your skin.

The more you practice gratitude, the happier you will feel. And, in time, you might even find gratitude for challenging things, like PCOS. Could you be grateful for the opportunity it has given you to learn about your body? Do you see how you can turn things around from dark to light? This is how gratitude becomes a powerful tool against depression and negative thinking.

Digital Detox

There has never been a time in history when technology has dominated our lives, social circles, and minds as much as now. Think about the time you spend looking at a screen. The average person spends around 5 hours a day on their phone. You might be reading this book on it now! But it isn't just phones. It's televisions, computers, tablets, laptops, billboards. We are ultra-connected, to our social media, to our smart homes, to our virtual lives. Unsurprisingly, this constant connection isn't doing our brains any good. We need time to switch off.

The rise of digital detox and mindfulness retreats shows just how many people are beginning to realize that we don't need digital connection to be happy. Sometimes it is beneficial to take time for ourselves and our loved ones without feeling the need to post it all over social media.

I would argue that social media doesn't do much for our happiness levels as we would like to think! We now have even more people to compare ourselves to, we are obsessed with the lives of people we have never met, and there is always a meme or three to point out something that we are not spending enough time on. We are bombarded by online tutorials teaching us everything from how to apply the perfect eyeliner to how to make the best vegan snacks. It is exhausting.

Let's consider what that smartphone is actually doing. It's like your own perfectly designed anxiety device that just sits in your pocket and demands your attention hundreds of times a day, mostly for meaningless reasons. The notifications trigger the part of our brain that deals with reactions to unknown and sudden external stimuli. The same part of the brain that deals with the fight or flight response. This leads to excess cortisol, which impacts the rest of your body. Your heart rate quickens, your chest tightens, and your palms get sweaty. Not just once a day, but multiple times a day. Every time one of your friends posts a video, when someone likes your photo, when a complete stranger comments on a post you liked two weeks ago, when one of your fifteen online news subscriptions publishes a story.

It is little wonder that this leads to overwhelm. All those notifications to check, to respond to, or to ignore. Many of us have a stress reaction to our phones, even when these notifications are positive, for example a text from your loved one or a friend.

So what can you do? Getting rid of your smartphone is not an option, since these are now such an integral part of almost everything we do. However, you can be smart about your smartphone use. Simply reducing your usage and being more mindful about when you plug in will have significant positive impact on your stress levels. You will feel more relaxed, better able to focus, and you'll have more time to connect with those around you, like your partner. Here are my tips for your very own daily digital detox:

- Switch off non-essential notifications. Do you really need to know every time someone views your post, or when a new product is available?
- Commit to going phone-free for one to two hours before bedtime. You can let loved ones know you're doing this if you think they might worry they can't get in touch with you.
- Do not look at social media or emails first thing in the morning. Allow yourself to fully wake up and set your intention for the day before you connect.
- Be disciplined - don't use your phone as a distraction all the time. Learn to be without it. If you're in a queue or on a train or bored, why not practice mindfulness in that moment instead of playing Candy Crush?

Proper Sleep

We all know how we feel after a good night's sleep. Except most of us can barely remember, because we do not get enough hours of sleep or enough quality sleep. And when it comes to PCOS, that's bad news.

I often find that when I speak to women about their most challenging PCOS symptoms, sleep pattern disruption always ranks high on the list. This is interesting since PCOS in itself doesn't directly cause problems sleeping. Being overweight or obese can increase your risk of sleep apnea (a condition whereby a person stops breathing in their sleep), which, unsurprisingly, leads to poor quality sleep. That being said, sleep problems most often stem from what you do, think, eat and drink during the day.

Sleep is one of those sacred processes that we cannot do without, and when we do sleep, we have to try to do it properly! That means sleeping long enough (between 7 and 9 hours) and getting enough time in the REM stage. This is when your brain detoxes and your body goes into repair mode. In Chapter 9, you'll find more details on sleep and how to make your night-time and morning routines work for you.

2. The Beauty Myth

The second thing impacting the way we feel is society's obsession with beauty. Our mothers might have told us that we're beautiful no matter what, but magazines, social media, adverts, billboards, tv shows, popular culture all scream at us that unless we look slender and flawless, we are lacking.

Added to that burden are the negative thoughts that naturally occur when you have PCOS and struggle daily with symptoms you feel you can't control. For me, it was the feeling of "what is wrong with me" every time another colleague went off on maternity leave that pulled me down into a spiral of self-hate. In a 2010 study carried out by the Selcuk University Faculty of Psychiatry, researchers compared women suffering from PCOS with healthy women and found that those with PCOS experienced lower self-esteem and had a more negative view of themselves and their bodies compared with healthy women.

You might think that this is normal. Most women will put themselves down for their looks, their weight, their age, their fertility. But this constant self-criticism is destructive. Thoughts might not be tangible things, but they none the less change your body. We saw earlier how stress (your thoughts about a situation) triggers physical changes (higher levels of cortisol, faster heart-rate etc.). When you constantly criticize yourself or view yourself with hate, your body responds. In fact, some studies have found a correlation between negative emotions such as anger or self-hate and immune diseases (conditions where the body's immune system turns on itself - which is basically a physical manifestation of self-hate).

So it is imperative that you begin to love your body. I know it's hard. We have not been taught how to do this. In fact, sometimes it feels as though society keeps us insecure so that we keep buying make up and clothes and products in a bid to make ourselves look and feel ok. These days, self-love is practically an act of rebellion. It is saying: no matter my size, no matter my current struggles, no matter my looks, I love me.

This is a journey that you must go on. Without self-love, the dietary and lifestyle changes you make will only get you so far. Here is a list of hacks to begin stepping out of that self-critical mindset and into loving yourself.

- Focus on what you love: We all have bits of our bodies that we dislike and we tend to focus on those so much that we lose sight of anything else. Find a part of your body that you find attractive. Anything at all. When I began this process, all I loved was my pinky finger! This process starts chipping away at the habitual criticism and turns your mindset towards appreciation for your body.
- Ask for help: Sometimes we find it hard to see the beauty in us, physical and mental. So, ask your friends and loved ones what they love about you. Listen with an open heart and let the words sink in. You can even write them down and look back at them next time you feel down about yourself.
- Be your own best friend: If we had a person in our life who said to us the things that we say to ourselves, that person would not be our friend! When you look in the mirror, speak to yourself as though you're speaking to your best friend. Tell yourself how great that dress looks on, how bright your eyes are, how well that color goes with your skin tone. The more love and appreciation you can show yourself, the more that will shine into all areas of your life.

3. Diet and Depression

We have briefly touched on diet as one of the big factors in PCOS. Interestingly, the foods that causes hormonal imbalances also increase your risk of depression. The two main culprits here are an excess of sugar and the wrong kinds of fat.

Sugar, which is present in almost all pre-made foods and drinks, triggers the same parts of the brain as hard drugs like cocaine. It stimulates the release of dopamine (a feel-good neurochemical, one of the main elements in drug highs - and the reason eating cake makes us feel good), and this has led scientists to conclude that sugar is an addictive substance that causes withdrawal symptoms, binging and depression. The more sugar you eat, the higher your likelihood of feeling low. Sugar increases inflammation. Studies have shown that high levels of inflammatory cytokines are involved in mood disorders like depression and anxiety.

We are eating more sugar than ever before, with average consumption at around 150g of the white stuff a day. Little wonder that waistlines have exploded and mental health is at an all-time low. Giving up sugar might sound scary, but trust me - it is easier than you think. The trick is to choose new foods that will satisfy your sweet tooth without spiking your insulin or increasing your levels of inflammation. You'll find a list of alternatives in Chapter 7.

Another thing increasing our mood disorders is the lack of healthy fats in our diets. Back in the 80's, fat became enemy #1 and everyone went fat-free. The theory was that saturated fat increased bad cholesterol and the risk of heart disease. This completely ignored the fact that the brain needs fat to function properly, and that female hormonal production depends on healthy fats. Now, we know better. Only a small part of the cholesterol in your blood comes from food - most of it is made by the body, usually in response to inflammation. So there is no need to be afraid of fat - rather, it's important to choose the right kinds of fat that will feed your brain, support your body and balance your hormones. That means avoiding trans-fats (like hydrogenated or partially hydrogenated oils) and certain vegetable oils (like canola, safflower, sunflower), which are too high in Omega-6 fatty acids and therefore inflammatory. It's easy to do this, simply by avoiding processed foods, fast foods and fried junk foods. Instead, focus on healthy fats from nuts and seeds. You'll find a list of healthy fats in Chapter 7.

In the previous chapter I mentioned that SSRI's are commonly prescribed for mood disorders. Unfortunately, they don't work that well, and come with the risk of serious side effects. But did you know that certain foods can boost your levels of serotonin naturally? Your body actually produces its own serotonin. To do so, it needs a particular amino acid called tryptophan. You can boost your levels of serotonin by including some of these tryptophan-rich foods in your daily diet:

- Pumpkin seeds
- Chia seeds
- Sesame seeds
- Sunflower seeds
- Soy beans and tofu
- Oats and oat bran
- Wheat germ

- Buckwheat
- White beans
- Pinto beans
- Kidney beans
- Black beans
- Lentils

By avoiding the foods that are proven to increase depression, you can begin to balance your mood while also reducing inflammation and therefore giving your body the best chance to overcome PCOS.

You now know how to tackle two of the biggest players when it comes to low mood: stress, and low self-esteem. We've briefly looked at how your diet impacts your mood and some of the foods that can help fight this, and we'll go into more detail about what foods to eat to heal PCOS in Chapter 7. If you're feeling overwhelmed, stop and take a deep breath now. You do not need to implement every single change right this second. And please don't feel guilty that you have many elements of your life to change. PCOS did not happen overnight, so healing it will take time - you can begin today simply by choosing one or two of the strategies suggested in this chapter and putting them into practice.

Before we get to the best foods and dietary practices to heal PCOS, I want to talk about fertility - if you're not trying to conceive, you can skip the next chapter and jump straight to Chapter 7.

CHAPTER SIX:

YOUR FERTILITY

We have now looked into the causes and symptoms of PCOS, and some of the strategies you can begin to practice to improve your mood, lower inflammation, and banish all those unwanted symptoms. But if you are anything like me, this is the chapter you have been waiting for. From the moment I got my PCOS diagnosis, the only thing I could think was, *"But will I ever be able to get pregnant?"*

If you are in this situation right now, then I am delighted that I can help you with this part. The information out there can be confusing and contradictory, and it is incredibly frustrating to work your way through medical journals and research papers, with all their complex jargon and mile-long sentences. In this chapter, I want to present some of the biggest challenges we face in terms of fertility, and what you can do to redress the situation. I would recommend speaking to a functional doctor or holistic practitioner about your fertility as it is a fascinating and complex area. The information contained here will at least give you a solid foundation from which to continue your research.

Standard Treatments for Fertility

Many of the ways modern medicine tackles fertility are woeful.

One option is to take prescription drugs like Metformin (a drug usually prescribed to improve insulin sensitivity in diabetic patients). Since insulin resistance is a big factor in PCOS, better insulin sensitivity can stimulate menstrual cycles. Another drug on offer is Clomiphene, which stimulates ovulation. Neither of these drugs actually addresses the underlying problems causing PCOS or infertility. Insulin resistance is a problem caused by a high-sugar diet. And artificially stimulating ovulation with chemicals can lead to a host of problems, such as the risk of ovarian hyperstimulation syndrome (which can be life threatening), rapid weight gain, hot flashes, breast pain, depression and heavy periods.

If drugs don't work, a surgical procedure known as ovarian drilling may be suggested. Ovarian drilling is basically a keyhole surgery where small holes are drilled into the ovaries to help eggs to be released. While it can stimulate regular egg release for up to 12 months, this procedure does nothing to address the underlying hormonal imbalances that are causing PCOS in the first place.

Finally, IVF (in vitro fertilization) is an option if you have been on a fertility treatment journey for a while or are over the age of 40. It is possible to conceive naturally with PCOS, especially if you change your diet and lifestyle. However, past the age of 40 this can be more challenging since at this time most women naturally have fewer eggs, which can make it harder to conceive naturally. But it has to be said that IVF is not a miracle solution. It can be incredibly challenging, emotional, and, ultimately, there is always the chance that it will not work. To give it the best chances of being successful, you have to be as healthy as you can.

Interestingly, being as healthy as you can actually puts you in a much better position, not just to conceive naturally, but also to avoid any pregnancy complications associated with PCOS (like gestational diabetes and the risk of needing a caesarian section). The strategies in this book into practice will help you get started on that journey.

Pregnancy Is Possible

Before we dive into the main risk factors for fertility, I want to tell you that there is hope. Having a child, despite PCOS, *is* possible and there are many success stories of women who have achieved this. As more lifestyle and wellness solutions to minimizing the symptoms of PCOS become apparent, there is growing evidence that these changes can have a positive effect on fertility as well. Modern medicine is now aware of this. In the absence of an actual cure for PCOS, medical professionals are more willing to recommend courses of treatment that include regular exercise, stress-relieving activities, and changes in your diet. This is because we are becoming aware of how important our overall lifestyle, diet, and mental health are to our physical health. And fertility is just one example of this relationship.

When I was struggling with my diagnosis, I found great comfort in stories like that of Chiara Ferragni, who bravely posted on Instagram about her struggles with PCOS. When she was able to conceive, I began to feel hopeful about my own situation. Seeing stories like that on social media is important. Remember that your body responds to your thoughts. If you believe that PCOS means you will never get pregnant, constantly reinforcing that idea may end up producing that exact intended outcome. I'm not saying that simply believing you can get pregnant will result in pregnancy, but you can help your body to welcome that state by thinking of yourself as able to carry a new life into the world. The first step to overcoming fertility issues is to visualize yourself as a healthy, glowing, loving mother.

What's Impacting Your Fertility?

Unsurprisingly, some of the risk factors in PCOS are the same risk factors in infertility.

1. Being overweight or underweight:

Being overweight affects hormone production and impacts ovarian function, making it harder to conceive. If you are underweight, there is not enough body fat to produce enough sex hormones, and this too impacts your fertility.

You are more likely to conceive if you are within your ideal weight range - that means a BMI of between 19 and 24.

Forget dieting - you can achieve a healthy weight simply by swapping processed foods for home-cooked alternatives and favoring whole foods, and including some exercise in your daily routine. The next two chapters will go into more detail about this.

2. Chemicals

We're in contact with more man-made chemicals than ever before - and it's making it increasingly hard to get pregnant. In a ground-breaking study, scientists discovered a link between persistent environmental pollutants and fertility problems. They identified fifteen chemicals: nine PCBs (polychlorinated biphenyls - used as cooling fluids in electricals), which have been banned for decades but are still present in the environment; three pesticides; two types of phthalates (a type of plastic found in personal care products and plastic containers), and furan, a toxic by-product from industrial combustion. The couples who were exposed to higher levels of these chemicals had more trouble conceiving. It's worth mentioning here that there are thousands of new chemicals released onto the market every year, but due to lack of funding, their effects on health are not studied.

A special mention should be made of pesticides, in particular glyphosate, which is the most widely used chemical in agriculture. Glyphosate is bad news for your health. It has been shown to disrupt your gut health, leading to digestive disorders, leaky gut, and higher levels of inflammation. Inflammation, as we know, increases your risk of PCOS. It has also been linked to cancer (as confirmed in August 2018, when a court ruled that Monsanto, the makers of glyphosate, had caused a man's lymphoma).

But I don't say that to scare you. We can't do much about the air quality, or what comes through the tap. But you can reduce your exposure to many chemicals simply by choosing different foods and different products.

- Avoid plastics as much as you can:
    o Use a glass or steel water bottle and coffee-cup.
    o Replace your plastic Tupperware with glass, steel or ceramic containers.
    o Avoid take-out cups as these are lined with plastic.
    o Never cook or microwave food in a plastic container.
- If the ingredients list sounds like a science experiment, leave that product on the shelf.
- Switch to organic as much as you can - check out the Environmental Working Group's lists below. The Clean 15 refers to produce with lower levels of pesticide residues, and can be bought non-organic; the Dirty Dozen refers to produce with very high levels of pesticide residues, and should always be bought organic.
- Swap conventional household cleaners for plant-based natural alternatives - browse your local health food shop for options.
- Shop for natural, cruelty-free, organic skincare.

Clean 15 (you can buy these non-organic):

- Avocado
- Sweetcorn (buy organic to avoid GMO sweetcorn)
- Pineapple
- Onions
- Papaya (buy organic to avoid GMO papaya)
- Sweet frozen peas
- Eggplant
- Asparagus
- Cauliflower
- Cantaloupe melon
- Broccoli
- Mushrooms
- Cabbage
- Honeydew melon
- Kiwi

Dirty Dozen (buy these organic):

- Strawberries
- Spinach
- Kale
- Nectarines
- Apples
- Grapes
- Peaches
- Pears

- Tomatoes
- Celery
- Potatoes
- Hot peppers

3. Smoking & Drinking

Smoking isn't just bad for your lungs, it's terrible for your chances of conception. Cigarette smoke disrupts hormones and damages DNA, so much so that it can even affect the fertility of your future children. If you're still smoking, it's a good idea to quit now and give yourself and your baby the best chance of health.

While drinking in moderation (less than one drink a day) isn't a problem, heavy drinking is linked with an increased risk of ovulation disorders. In fact, women who are heavy drinkers are more likely to seek fertility treatment. Stick with organic wines or spirits and keep sugar-heavy beers and cocktails to a minimum.

4. Oral and Injectable Contraceptives

We briefly touched on the problem with contraceptives earlier in the book. It seems obvious that a pharmaceutical designed to stop you conceiving will impact on your future chances of conceptions - at least for the time it takes for your body to readjust to its natural hormone levels.

Contraceptives are usually a combination of estrogen and progesterone. They work by stopping the release of luteinizing hormone and follicle stimulating hormone - these are the hormones responsible for releasing the egg and preparing the uterus for the fertilized egg to develop. Progesterone thickens the mucus around the egg, making it harder to fertilize,

But taking synthetic hormones stops your body producing the hormones it needs to. That means that it will take time for your body to return to balance. Because contraceptives are often prescribed as a way of regulating the menstrual cycle, many women go for years not knowing their own hormones are out of balance. Only when they want to start a family and come off the pill do these problems become more apparent.

A great way to reconnect with your cycle is to monitor it. As suggested earlier, you can do this in a journal. There are also digital family planning apps, like Natural Cycles (Cyclerpedia), that help you to get in touch with your period. It works by using your morning temperature to ascertain where you are in your cycle and whether you are ovulating or not, which will help you and your partner if you are trying to conceive. If you choose to see a fertility specialist, this information will be of interest to them.

Now that we've looked at the factors involved in fertility, it's time to discuss what a hormone-friendly lifestyle looks like. In the next two chapters, we'll look at the key areas in your life where you can make a change. I'm going to guide you through how to transform your diet and your exercise routine.

CHAPTER SEVEN:

YOUR FOOD IS YOUR MEDICINE

It's been said so much that it's a cliché, but that doesn't make it any less true: You are what you eat. With PCOS, this could not be more accurate. When I first learned about the impact of my diet on my symptoms, I have to admit I was skeptical. I didn't really want to believe it because I didn't really want to change. Food is such an integral part of our everyday lives that to overhaul years of habits, misinformation, and ignorance is quite a task.

Thankfully we now live in a digital age, where information is quite literally at our fingertips. But this can lead to information overload. I mean, who do you believe when there are so many competing schools of thought? When it comes to PCOS, there are certain accepted points, such as the need to reduce sugar, but there is not much consensus on anything else. With all these opinions, it can be difficult to know what changes to make. And this can lead to you not making any change at all.

Allow me to demystify healthy living. It is not about following someone else's strict dietary protocol, but rather about finding the foods that suit you and your tastes. By listening to your body and how it responds to various foods and situations (and this is where the journaling is invaluable) you can create your very own health protocol. And that is going to be much easier to stick to than someone else's rules!

That said, there are some basic rules to healthy living. We've already looked at why you'll need to remove refined sugar and processed foods from your life... but what do you need to include on your plate?

And how are you going to switch from buying pre-made foods, to making your meals from scratch?

These are the questions that will be answered in this chapter.

What Makes a Healthy Diet?

A healthy diet consists of a good balance of macronutrients and micronutrients. Macronutrients are the nutrients you need in large quantities: carbohydrates, proteins and fats. Micronutrients are nutrients you need in small quantities: vitamins, minerals, and antioxidants.

Our western diets are much too high in refined carbohydrates and bad fats, while being woefully low in vitamins and minerals. As a result, we are malnourished and sick. It is time to redress that.

Carbohydrates

These are your body's preferred source of energy. Your digestive system breaks down carbohydrates into glucose, which your cells can then use as fuel. In PCOS, the issue is that we're eating too many refined carbohydrates, which then trigger high levels of insulin to be released, and, over time, insulin resistance, weight gain and hormonal problems.

Refined carbohydrates are basically whole grains that have been processed to remove the germ and the husk, leaving only the starch. In other words, the protein, fat and fiber have been removed. This means there is nothing to slow down the absorption of sugar. Result: insulin spikes and insulin resistance. Complex carbohydrates, on the other hand, contain fiber and other nutrients. They take longer for your body to break down, resulting in lower levels of insulin and better blood sugar control. The fiber they contain also helps keep you fuller for longer, so you end up snacking less.

Carbohydrates are not the enemy, even though some dietary protocols advocate not eating any (paleo and ketogenic diets restrict daily carbohydrates to under 50 grams per day). The trick is the choose the right kinds of carbohydrates. Ones that supply your body with fuel, but also contain nutrients that prevent your blood sugar from going haywire.

One example is fruit. Some say fruit is bad for you because it contains sugar. What those people forget is that this naturally occurring sugar is accompanied by fiber, water, and vitamins. And this means it has a completely different effect on your body and blood sugar compared to sweets, for example. So, while the sugar in fruit is a simple carbohydrate, fruit itself can be considered a source of complex carbohydrates.

- Simple carbohydrates:
  - Refined foods (white flour, white pasta, white rice, white bread), which are made from flours that have had the fiber removed.
  - Added sugars (cane sugar, high fructose corn syrup, honey, agave syrup…).
  - Naturally occurring sugars in fruit (fructose) and milk (lactose).
- Complex carbohydrates:
  - Fiber (found in vegetables, whole grains, beans, legumes, fruits)
  - Starch (found in whole grains, root vegetables and beans).

Refined Carbohydrates & Healthy Alternatives	
White bread	Wholegrain bread (spelt, buckwheat, kamut, barley, rye…) Wholegrain sourdough bread Wholegrain soda bread
White pasta / noodles / couscous	Wholegrain pasta Buckwheat pasta / buckwheat noodles Pasta made from beans and legumes like lentils, peas, or brown rice

Potato fries / crisps	Sweet potato wedges
	Roasted beetroot
	Celeriac fries
	Vegetable crisps (made from carrots, parsnips, beetroot, sweet potatoes)
Cakes, biscuits, pastries, sweets	Fresh fruit (pair it with a few nuts or seeds for slow & steady release of energy)
	Home-made fruit smoothie
	Home-made energy bar or flapjack
	Home-made high-fiber biscuits
	75-95% dark organic chocolate
	Home-made chocolate truffles

Gluten

Before we move onto protein, I'd like to say something about gluten, which is found in wheat, rye and barley. Should you avoid it? I would recommend cutting it out of your life for at least a month, just to see how your body reacts. Many people are either incredibly sensitive to gluten or only mildly sensitive - regardless, if there is some sensitivity, this means that in the background, gluten is contributing to chronic inflammation, which is the last thing you want when you're trying to heal PCOS.

Some scientists consider that the rise in autoimmune conditions and digestive disorders are due not so much to gluten, but rather to the glyphosate residues in the grain. This could indicate that you can continue eating it as long as you choose organic varieties, and as long as you are not sensitive to gluten.

My advice would be to listen to your body and record how it reacts after you eat gluten, and then cut it out of your diet for the first month. After that, slowly reintroduce it and see how you feel. Your body is always communicating with you, if you listen. If it turns out that you are sensitive to gluten, don't worry - this doesn't have to spell the end of all things delicious. There are plenty of gluten-free grains that are just as delicious, and even more nutritious.

Protein

Protein is an essential component of every single cell. Your body needs it to maintain your tissues and muscles.

When you read "protein", what's the first thing you think about? Most people will think of meat. The reason meat is considered the best source of protein is because it contains all nine essential amino acids (this makes meat a "complete" protein). These amino acids are called essential because the body cannot make them, and they therefore have to be obtained from food.

But meat is not the only complete protein out there, far from it. What's more, it is possible to combine plant foods to obtain all essential amino acids and form a complete protein.

Maybe you're thinking - who cares, I'm going to stick with

meat. Unfortunately, we are eating way too much meat these days. We have bacon for breakfast, chicken for lunch, steak for dinner. Not only is this having a dramatic and destructive impact on our planet, it is damaging our health. And that's without mentioning the cruelty involved in animal agriculture. I do not wish to preach - there are many people speaking out about this and they have more information than me on the topic. I would urge you to do some research. Cowspiracy, for example, exposes the environmental impact. Earthlings and Dominion expose the conditions animals have to endure before being turned into neat cellophaned packages in the supermarket aisle.

I've found that most people, once they are given the truth about how their food choices impact the planet and other conscious beings, either completely avoid or dramatically reduce their consumption of animal products. That was the case for me. Five years ago, I would have laughed in your face if you'd told me I'd be choosing beans over chicken nuggets. But once I experienced how much better I felt, not just in my body but in my heart. As a mum, I didn't want to be contributing to global destruction. I believe we all have a part to play in maintaining a safe and green planet for our children and grandchildren. Going vegan is one of the most powerful ways we can do that.

In terms of PCOS, avoiding animal products helps improve your symptoms. That's because meat and dairy have been proven to increase inflammation, while a plant-based diet actively lowers inflammation. If you can't go without meat completely, then at least aim to have a few meat-free days a week, and switch to organic, sustainably reared meat. Go to your local farmer's market and interact with producers, rather than buying from the supermarket. Independent, local producers are more likely to treat the animals with respect, and organically reared animals are not given tons of antibiotics, growth hormones, or feed containing animal remains and/or GMO grains.

Ok, but what about protein? Good news - you can get all the protein you need through plants. Below you'll find a list of all nine essential amino acids and the best food sources. The following plant foods are complete proteins:

- Buckwheat
- Soy beans (edamame, tofu, tempeh)
- Hemp seeds
- Chia seeds
- Quinoa
- Spirulina

You can also combine foods that contain different amino acids to obtain all nine:

- Grains with beans or legumes (for example: peanut butter on oat crackers, rice and lentils, kidney beans and millet).
- Seeds or nuts with beans or legumes (for example: sunflowers seeds with black beans, Chickpeas and sesame seeds (hummus), pumpkin seeds and mung beans).

Plant Sources of Essential Amino Acids

Histidine	Isoleucine	Leucine*	Lysine*	Methionine	Phenylalanine	Threonine	Tryptophan	Valine
Tofu	Tofu	Tofu	Tofu	Tofu	Tofu	Tofu	Tofu	Tofu
Oats	Lupin beans	Oats	Edamame beans	Oats & oat bran	Edamame beans	Lupin beans	Oats	Oats
Buckwheat	Lentils	Navy beans	Green peas	Brazil nuts	Oats	Oats	Buckwheat	Buckwheat
Lentils	Oats & oat bran	Adzuki beans	Lupin beans	Teff grain	Navy beans	Buckwheat	Pumpkin seeds	Navy beans
White beans	Buckwheat	White beans	Navy beans	Wheat germ	Lupin beans	White beans	Sea vegetables	Lupin beans
Kidney beans	Lima beans	Buckwheat	Adzuki beans	Corn	White beans	Navy beans	Whole wheat	White beans
Adzuki beans	Chickpeas	Lentils	Lentils & lentil sprouts	Buckwheat	Kidney beans	Lentils	Walnuts	Oat bran
Mung beans	Swiss chard	Mung beans	White beans	Hemp seeds	Pinto beans	Adzuki beans	Lentils	Adzuki beans
Pea sprouts	Whole wheat pasta	Broad beans	Split peas	White beans	Buckwheat	Split peas	Mung beans	Lentils and lentil sprouts
Wild rice / Chia seeds	Pistachios	Teff grain	Buckwheat	Kidney beans	Lentils and lentil sprouts	Corn	Chickpeas	Kidney beans
Almonds	Spinach	Kamut grain	Oats	Sesame seeds	Mung beans	Chickpeas	Chia seeds	Lima beans
Sunflower seeds	Wild rice	Pumpkin seeds	Black beans	Lentils	Cornmeal	Soy sprouts	Sesame seeds	Black beans
Whole wheat pasta	Quinoa	Hemp seeds	Mung beans	Green peas	Hemp seeds	Black eyed peas	Sunflower seeds	Peanuts
Peanuts	Sunflower seeds	Spirulina	Quinoa	Sweet potato	Peanuts	Broad beans	Quinoa	Flax seeds
			Hemp seeds	Millet	Quinoa	Teff grain	Potatoes	Brown rice
					Sunflower seeds	Hemp seeds	Pine nuts	Spinach
					Millet	Wheat-germ		Cashew nuts
					Almonds	Pumpkin seeds		
						Peanuts		

Dairy

While we're on the topic of alternatives to animal products, let me talk about dairy for a moment. Dairy is particularly problematic when it comes to PCOS because it contains a particular protein that spikes insulin levels - casein. Studies show that a glass of milk can increase insulin levels higher and faster than a slice of white bread. It also increases inflammation and messes with your hormones.

The toxins and antibiotic residues in conventional cow's milk do not support or enhance the human digestive system. They actually cause digestive issues, which in turn can trigger immune responses. Most people do not have adequate levels of lactase (the digestive enzyme responsible for breaking down and digesting lactose, the sugar in milk) after childhood. This leads to symptoms such as bloating, excess mucus, and even acne. If you want to lower your levels of inflammation, keep your insulin levels under control, and help alleviate symptoms like acne, then it's time to show dairy the door.

When I first thought about going vegan, there were very few plant-based options. These days, you are spoilt for choice. Just remember to check the label and go for organic varieties with no added sugars and no ingredients that you can't pronounce!

Fats

As we saw earlier, fat is not the enemy. In fact, it is essential for normal hormonal function. However, the quality of fat is important. Animal fats have been linked to higher levels of inflammation, as have hydrogenated fats and some vegetable oils. On the other hands, certain plant sources fats have been linked to lower levels of inflammation and improved mood.

Fats to Avoid	Healthy fats to Include
Trans fats:	**Oils:**
Hydrogenated vegetable oils	Coconut oil
Partially hydrogenated vegetable oils	Extra virgin olive oil
Margarine	Avocado oil
Shortening	Flaxseed oil
Red meat	Walnut oil
Full fat dairy (cream, butter, ghee)	
	Whole foods:
	Nuts
Vegetable oils:	Seeds
Canola oil	Avocados
Rapeseed oil	
Soy oil	
Corn oil	
Sunflower oil	

Micronutrients

Vitamins, minerals, antioxidants. But what does that even mean? These are the compounds that help every part of the body to function. They are essential for health. Without them, we get sick. For example, without adequate vitamin C, the immune system cannot function properly. Without adequate magnesium, bones can go brittle. Without B vitamins, cells struggle to produce energy from food. It would take a whole other book to go into all the various functions of all the vitamins available to us.

Fruits, vegetables, whole grains, nuts, seeds - these are nature's medicine cabinet. All whole foods contain a variety of vitamins, minerals, and antioxidants. But these compounds are delicate - deep fry a potato and all the vitamin C it contains disappears (not to mention the added health burden of the vegetable oil needed to fry it). Your ready meal might contain vegetables, but that doesn't mean it contains vitamins - after all, they are also packed with sugar, chemicals, and preservatives, wrapped in plastic, and then stored in warehouses and supermarket shelves for weeks or months.

All this to say that the best way to get enough vitamins, minerals and antioxidants is simply to eat whole foods, and to prepare them yourself. Below, you'll find a table showing essential vitamins and where to find them. This is just a guide rather than an exhaustive list, and I hope it shows you how many micronutrients are present in plant foods, and how varied your diet can be. You don't need to eat one food from each list (and indeed, you'll find some of the foods contain various vitamins) every day, just try to include a variety of whole foods in your diet. If you fill at least half your plate with fresh vegetables, you'll be giving yourself plenty of micronutrients.

Before we go on, a word on antioxidants. Antioxidants are, as the name implies, compounds that stop oxidation. Oxidation happens in the body in response to pollutants and other toxins (also known as free radicals). Quick science: free radicals are molecules that are missing an electron, and therefore unstable. They go around the body stealing electrons from other molecules, thereby turning those molecules into free radicals, and on it goes. Antioxidants are able to donate an electron, thereby neutralizing the free radicals and halting any further damage. Oxidation is a risk factor in inflammation and therefore PCOS, so foods that actively stop that process are going to go a long way to helping alleviate your symptoms.

Where can you find them? Fresh fruits and vegetables, especially brightly colored ones. There are hundreds of antioxidants, but three of these deserve a special mention, because they have been studied in relation to their anti-inflammatory potential. They are anthocyanidin, quercetin and chlorophyll. All three can help lower your levels of inflammation, and are therefore well worth adding to your PCOS healing protocol.

Quercetin	Anthocyanidin	Chlorophyll
Capers	Eggplant	Spinach
Red onions	Black beans	Parsley
Black plums	Blackberries	Kelp
Blueberries	Blueberries	Beet tops
Cherries	Cherries	Turnip tops
Cranberries	Elderberries	Leafy greens (kale, collard greens, arugula)
Hot green chili peppers	Nectarines	
	Plums	
Red leaf lettuce	Radishes	Asparagus
Kale	Raspberries	Green pepper
Buckwheat	Red apples	Green beans
Elderberries	Red cabbage	Spirulina
Cacao	Red kidney beans	Chlorella
Dill	Red onion	
Tarragon	Red or black grapes	
Cilantro	Strawberries	
Red apples		

Vitamin A	Vitamin C	Vitamin E	Vitamin B1	Vitamin B3
Apricots	Broccoli	Beans	Asparagus	Almonds
Asparagus	Cabbage	Almonds	Beans	Asparagus
Broccoli	Cauliflower	Brazil nuts	Brazil nuts	Cabbage
Cabbage	Collard	Hazelnuts	Brussels	Cauliflower
Carrots	greens	Oily fish	Sprouts	Chia seeds
Collard	Grapefruit	Peanuts	Cabbage	Zucchini
greens	Kiwis	Peas	Cashew	Eggs
Mangoes	Lemons	Pecans	nuts	Mushrooms
Melon	Lime	Quinoa	Cauliflower	Squash
Papayas	Melon	Sesame	Chia seed	Tempeh
Pumpkin	Oranges	seeds	Zucchini	Tomatoes
Squash	Peas	Sunflower	Lettuce	Whole
Sweet	Peppers	seeds	Mushrooms	wheat
potatoes	Strawberries	Sweet	Peas	
Tangerines	Tomatoes	potatoes	Pecans	
Tomatoes	Watercress	Wheatgerm	Peppers	
Watercress			Squash	
			Tomatoes	
			Watercress	

Vitamin B6	Biotin	Choline	Calcium	Chromium
Asparagus	Almonds	Collard greens	Tofu	Broccoli
Banana	Sweet potatoes	Good quality multivitamin supplement	Sesame seeds	Barley
Broccoli	Onions		Collard greens	Oats
Brussels sprouts	Oats		Spinach	Green beans
Cabbage	Tomatoes		Turnip greens	Tomatoes
Cashew nuts	Peanuts		Mustard greens	Romaine lettuce
Cauliflower	Carrots		Beet greens	
Dates	Walnuts			
Hazelnuts				
Lentils				
Onions				
Peppers				
Red kidney beans				
Seeds and nuts				
Squash				
Tempeh				
Watercress				

Iodine	Iron	Magnesium	Manganese	Selenium
Sea salad	Soy beans	Pumpkin seeds	Oats	Brazil nuts
Kelp	Lentils	Spinach	Brown rice	Cabbage
Wakame	Spinach	Swiss chard	Chickpeas	Chia seeds
Nori	Sesame seeds	Soy beans	Spinach	Zucchinis
Dulse	Chickpeas	Sesame seeds	Pineapple	Molasses
	Lima beans	Black beans	Pumpkin seeds	Mushrooms
	Olives	Quinoa	Rye	
	Navy beans	Cashew nuts	Tempeh	
	Swiss chard	Sunflower seeds	Soy beans	
	Kidney beans	Beet greens		

Zinc	Potassium	Vitamin D3	Vitamin B12
Sesame seeds	Beet greens	Mushrooms	Nutritional yeast
Pumpkin seeds	Sweet potato	Fortified plant milks	Fortified plant milks
Lentils	Swiss chard	Good quality Vitamin D supplement	Good quality B12 supplement
Chickpeas	Potatoes		
Cashew nuts	Lima beans		
Quinoa	Spinach		
	Bok choy		
	Beetroot		
	Brussels sprouts		

The important thing to remember is that any short-term discomfort of changing your diet will be outweighed by being able to live a life where you are free from PCOS, your weight is under control, and you have increased levels of happiness. If it all feels too much, simply begin with one small step, for example decide that one meal a day will be completely plant-based and home-made. Over time, these small tweaks can build into lifelong positive change.

Low GI Foods

One of the most commonly prescribed diets for PCOS is a low-GI diet. GI stands for glycemic index, which ranks foods based on impact they have on your blood sugar. The lower a food's GI, the less insulin needs to be produced, so this diet is extremely effective for PCOS sufferers. The GI scale can help you distinguish between healthy and unhealthy carbs.

The GI Scale is divided into three sections: low (GI 55 or less), medium (GI 56-59) and high (GI 70 or more).

Several factors go into determining a food's glycemic index, including the structure of the starch, the type of sugar present, and how refined the food is. Food preparation, cooking methods, and ripeness can also have an influence on the number.

While using a food's GI can be helpful, it isn't the be-all-and-end-all. The thing to bear in mind as well is that how a food affects your insulin levels will also depend on the foods it is paired with. For example, just having a piece of fruit will trigger a higher insulin spike than if you have that piece of fruit with a handful of nuts - that's because the protein, fiber and fat in the nuts slows down the breakdown of glucose and leads to lower levels of insulin having to be released.

PCOS Superfoods

As you can see, improving your overall diet in relation to PCOS is simply about replacing processed, high sugar foods with the right organic whole, home-cooked foods (don't worry if you don't think you have the time - the next section will explore how you can make time in your schedule for food prep). Having said that, some foods are superfoods. Health professionals widely agree that eating these foods is good for your health, but because of their specific properties, they are doubly beneficial for PCOS sufferers.

Avocados:

Well known for being brain-friendly, the avocado is a great source of Omega 3 fatty acids (which fight inflammation) and Vitamin E (a powerful antioxidant), both of which are fantastic for giving the skin a healthy glow. The presence of healthy fats can help balance hormones, as well as regulate blood sugar. All in all, well-deserving of number one spot on our superfood list! Mash up into a guacamole, blend with cacao to make a chocolate mousse, or spoon onto sourdough toast for a healthy breakfast.

Berries:

Low in sugar and packed with antioxidants, berries are your best friend in your crusade against PCOS. Throw them in a smoothie or add them to overnight oats for a touch of sweetness that won't spike your blood sugar.

Nuts and seeds:

Great for healthy snacking and regulating sugar levels, a handful of nuts will also help to reduce androgen levels and cholesterol. Seeds such as flax seeds and chia seeds contain fiber that helps keep you regular and stabilize hormone levels.

Legumes and beans:

The importance of fiber cannot be understated, particularly when obtained from healthy sources such as vegetables and legumes. Fiber slows down the absorption of sugar, which helps combat insulin resistance. The fiber also feeds the good bacteria in your gut, and a healthy gut means a healthy immune system and lower inflammation. Legumes are a fantastic combination of both protein and fiber, which helps you to feel fuller for longer and curb cravings, so they can help you lose weight.

Ok, so now you know the right foods to include, how does this look in practice? The thing to remember is to obtain a balance of nutrients:

- 2 or more cups of antioxidant-rich foods
- Complex carbohydrates

- Plant sources of protein
- Plant sources of healthy fats

Here is an example of how this could look:

Meals	Nutrients
Breakfast: Blueberry smoothie and overnight oats with hemp seeds	Antioxidants (berries) Healthy fats (hemp seeds) Omega 3 (hemp seed)
Lunch: Quinoa salad with arugula, avocado, peppers, tomatoes, tahini & turmeric dressing	Healthy fats (avocado, tahini) Antioxidants & micronutrients (arugula, peppers, turmeric) Plant protein and complex carbs (quinoa)
Dinner: Stir-fried broccoli, mushrooms & leeks with marinated tofu and buckwheat noodles	Antioxidants & micronutrients (broccoli, mushrooms, leeks) Plant protein and complex carbs (tofu, buckwheat)
Snack: Peanut, oat & coconut energy balls	Plant protein (peanut & oats combined) Healthy fats (coconut oil)

It is important to remember that this is not a diet in the traditional sense of the word. Your main goal is to re-nourish your body and rebalance your hormones, the weight loss will happen naturally. So, don't restrict your portions - doing this will only make you more likely to revert to bad habits. If you feel hungry, eat. But eat whole foods. When you eat nutrient-dense food as opposed to processed food (which is devoid of nutrients and leaves you feeling hungry), your appetite will normalize.

Another thing you will also notice is that your taste-buds change. When you eat processed foods, you get your taste-buds used to extreme sweetness and extreme saltiness. This leads you to crave those foods, and natural foods taste bland by comparison. However, just give yourself a week of eating clean, unprocessed foods, and you will find that your taste buds begin to appreciate the subtle sweetness in coconut and the savory flavor of toasted seeds - and you will begin craving those types of food instead.

Kitchen Preparation

Let's explore the changes you need to make to ensure you and your kitchen are fully prepared for your new healthy lifestyle.

How ready is your kitchen for the dietary overhaul that you are about to undertake? New meals mean new cooking methods, so your pantry needs to be fully stocked up with the right ingredients. Most healthy cookbooks contain information about the appliances or equipment you will need, but below you'll find my short list of essentials.

Blender:

Perfect for making the smoothest smoothies, and even healthy ice cream. Smoothies are a fantastic way to eat plenty of vegetables without having to chew your way through a huge bowlful. Simply put a couple of handfuls of greens in your blender and voila - green goodness. Of course, you can add a banana or apple to make it more palatable, or even add things like ginger and turmeric.

I prefer blenders over juicers, because with blenders you keep all the healthy fiber from the fruits and vegetables, which is essential for blood sugar control and will help keep you full until your next meal.

Slow Cooker:

Few things are better than a home-cooked meal after a hard day at work. Unfortunately, by the time we get home, cooking is the last thing that we want to be doing! But with a slow cooker, you can simply throw in your ingredients (chopped vegetables, beans, grains, spices, chopped tomatoes, etc.) and it will cook them up into a nutritious, tasty meal that's ready for when you finish work.

Steamer:

Vegetables can be cooked in a number of ways, but steaming is the best way to retain as many of their vitamins as possible. A steamer is also handy for saving you time, because it allows you to cook several vegetables at once. If steamed vegetables don't appeal to you, here's a chef trick: season them. Dressings are the best way to liven up steamed veg. It could be olive oil and lemon juice with chopped herbs and seeds, or tamari sauce and peanut butter, or tahini and turmeric - whatever flavors you enjoy.

Healthy Pantry

If your kitchen is full of unhealthy foods, you will be more likely to revert to bad habits. If you're really ready to take your health into your hands, then it's time to stock your kitchen with ingredients that enable you to throw together a healthy tasty meal in minutes. Here is a list to get you started. You don't need to get everything at once, the important thing is to begin.

Spices & Herbs	Grains	Legumes
Cumin	Brown rice	Chickpeas
Turmeric	Brown rice pasta	Black beans
Garam masala	Buckwheat	Cannellini beans
Chermoula	Buckwheat noodles	Red or brown lentils
Italian herb mix	Quinoa	Kidney beans
Curry powder	Millet	Black eye beans
Black pepper	Amaranth	Split peas
Paprika	Polenta	Mung beans
Oregano	Oats	(You can buy these dried or tinned for convenience)
Rosemary		
Baking	**Nuts & Seeds**	**Oils & Seasoning**
Buckwheat flour	Pumpkin seeds	Coconut oil
Rice flour	Sunflower seeds	Olive oil
Spelt flour	Chia seeds	Avocado oil
Kamut flour	Flax seeds	Sesame oil
Coconut flour	Almonds	Tamari sauce
Ground almonds	Hazelnuts	Apple cider vinegar
Dates	Brazil nuts	Himalayan salt

Apricots	Cashew nuts	Tinned tomatoes
Cacao butter	Coconut flakes	Tomato puree
Cacao powder	Tahini	
Vanilla powder	Peanut butter	
Cinnamon	Almond butter	

Making Time for Home-cooking

Once you're ready with some basic healthy ingredients, you're ready to get started… but there's a saying: "failing to plan is planning to fail."

This is particularly true when it comes to lifestyle changes. In order to successfully switch to a healthy diet, you must plan ahead. Make time in your schedule, set aside a couple of hours, and think about what you are going to eat for breakfast, lunch and dinner in the week ahead. Prepare for your grocery shop by thinking about the recipes and number of meals you will be cooking, so you can work out how much of each food you need.

Then, take a look at your diary and identify when you have time to batch-cook meals.

For example, at the weekend you could make enough soup, curry, or pasta bake for 3 or 4 meals and freeze individual portions. You could also pre-cook grains and make some salad dressings so that you can make a tasty salad for lunch in under 10 minutes. You could make overnight oats or chia pots in advance and have breakfast ready for 2 to 3 days.

Preparing food in advance means that on the days when you're too busy or exhausted to cook, all you need to do is grab a healthy home cooked meal out of the fridge or freezer and heat it up. This makes it much easier to stick to healthy habits.

I usually spend Sunday doing my grocery shopping, cooking and meal prepping, portioning out into containers to store in the refrigerator or freezer depending on when I plan to eat them. At the start, I found that there was a lot of leftover food, and it was hard to justify the much larger budget required for all the healthy components of that meal. But when I started portioning out food for the week, making more meals with fewer ingredients, and cooking for the whole family instead of just myself, I found that my leftovers reduced, and my average spending actually decreased.

Smoothies, broths and soups are excellent ways to use leftovers. Whatever vegetables you don't use for your evening meal can be thrown into your blender with a banana and some ginger root for breakfast. They can be boiled up into a vegetable broth that you can flavor with miso or herbs. Or they can form the base for a curry, stew, or vegetable lasagna. Make sure you have plenty of glass containers in your kitchen so you can store leftovers safely.

Breakfast

The most important thing in the morning is to make something as quickly and as healthy as possible. You want a breakfast that will give you energy and keep you satisfied till lunch. For that reason, smoothies, overnight oats, and chia pots are great options. At the weekend, or when you have more time to make something from scratch, why not experiment with scrambled tofu or banana pancakes?

Kale and Spinach Smoothie (serves 1)

Ingredients:

1 cup filtered water
1 cup chopped kale
1 cup chopped spinach
1 banana or 1 apple
1 tsp shaved ginger root

Throw it all in your blender, and blend at high speed until smooth. You can replace the water with ice cubes to make it colder and thicker. If it's too thick, add a little more water to dilute to your desired consistency.

Lunch

Lunch is your chance to refuel and give yourself the energy to power you through your afternoon, all the way till dinnertime. Think complex carbohydrates and healthy protein. Soups and salads are great options because you can easily get all your macronutrients: beans (protein), grains (complex carbs), vegetables (vitamins & antioxidants) and a dressing (healthy fats) and voila - a tasty lunch that is easy to carry to work in a jar.

Chickpea and Avocado Salad (serves 2)

Ingredients

1 cup cooked chickpeas
1 cup cooked quinoa (or other grain like rice)
2 avocados, chopped
1 cup romaine lettuce (or other leafy greens like spinach, arugula, watercress), roughly chopped
1 carrot, grated
2 sticks of celery, chopped
1 lemon, juiced
2 tbsp olive oil
Salt and pepper to taste

Cook the quinoa and chickpeas beforehand (it's a good idea to batch cook grains and beans so they're ready to be turned into a tasty meal in minutes).

Place all the ingredients in a large bowl and mix well to combine.

Store in the fridge, ready for when you need it. It will keep for 2-3 days in an airtight container.

Dinner

Whether you enjoy cooking like me or can think of nothing worse than going home and slaving over a hot stove, there are many healthy options that you can make with minimal cooking time. Try out this recipe for an evening meal that is easy to make during the week and is also a great crowd pleaser for when you have friends over.

Pea & Roots Curry (Serves 4-6)

Ingredients:

1 cup split peas
1 tbsp coconut oil (melted)
1 tsp curry powder
2 large beetroot (chopped)
2 sweet potato (chopped)
1 tsp coconut oil
1 onion (finely chopped)
1 thumb sized piece of ginger (grated)
1 thumb sized piece of turmeric (grated)
1 tbsp curry spice
3 sticks of celery (chopped)
1 handful of mushrooms (chopped)
2 cups vegetable stock
1 can full fat coconut cream
Pinch of salt

Soak the split peas overnight. Cook in a large pan with plenty of water for 40 minutes or until tender. Set aside.

In a large bowl, place the chopped beetroot and sweet potato, melted coconut oil and curry powder. Toss until evenly coated and place on a baking tray.

Roast in the oven at 400F for 20-30 minutes (the smaller the chunks, the less time this will take).

While the root veg is roasting, make the curry.

In a large saucepan, heat the coconut oil and fry the onion until translucent. Add the ginger and turmeric and fry for a minute, then add the curry powder and stir until the onion is coated and the spices release their fragrance.

Add the celery and mushrooms. Stir fry for a minute.

Add the stock and simmer for 3 minutes.

Add the coconut cream and split peas and cook for a further 5 minutes.

You can either mix the roasted vegetables into the curry or place the curry in a bowl and pile the roasted veg on top.

Serve with brown rice, quinoa, or buckwheat.

Snacks

Snacks don't have to be banished forever. But you need to approach snacking differently if you want overcome the symptoms of PCOS. As we discussed, sugar is a no-go area, so that means no sugary drinks, cookies, chocolate bars, and candy. This might be the hardest area to change, because many of us snack not out of hunger, but out of boredom.

That being said, sometimes you need that boost of energy between meals, especially if you are running errands all day. Here too, preparation is everything. Snacks that are available in the shops are, for the most part, packed with added sugar. Even healthier versions, like flap jacks, dried fruits, and trail mix can contain hidden sugar that will spike your insulin levels. If you make your own, you can snack guilt free, on foods that support your health instead of damaging it.

My favorite snacks are energy balls, simply because they are so quick to make and so versatile - especially if you have those pantry essentials in your cupboards.

Chocolate Peanut Energy Balls (makes 10-12 bites)

Ingredients:
1 cup smooth peanut butter (use unsalted and a brand made from 100% just peanuts)
1/3 cup dates, pitted
1/3 cup coconut flour
1/4 cup cacao powder

Place the ingredients in a food processor and process until the mixture is well combined.

Spoon a tablespoon of mixture into your hand and roll into a ball. Repeat with the rest of the mixture.

Place in the fridge to set for 2 hours.

Store in an airtight container in the fridge for 2 weeks.

Eating Out

No matter how prepared you are and how well you have stocked your pantry, you will, at some point, have to face eating out. After all, being healthy includes having a social life!

Thankfully, there are more and more restaurants offering not just vegan options, but healthy vegan options as well. Go on HappyCow.com and research what's around you. Choose a restaurant that has plenty of options, while also catering to your fellow diners. Don't be afraid to ask your friends for help choosing a venue that can cater to everyone's needs.

Finally, the thing to remember is… the 80-20 rule. Having a treat once in a while is ok. That's part of life. What matters is what you eat the majority of the time. So if you have dessert, it's ok. Don't beat yourself up about it, just make sure that you get back to your healthy habits the next day.

There you have it, you are now armed with the information to begin making positive changes to your diet that will reduce your insulin sensitivity, lower your inflammation, and begin healing PCOS.

CHAPTER EIGHT:
EXERCISE IS NON-NEGOTIABLE

Yes, you read that right. Exercise is *NON-negotiable*. Take a moment to let that sink in, and mourn your old couch potato life. There is no getting around the fact that you need to set aside time for exercise, at least 25-45 minutes every day, if you want to overcome your symptoms. Without daily exercise, the changes you make to your diet will only go so far. With exercise, you can speed up your healing process.

That said, please don't panic. Just because exercise is non-negotiable doesn't mean you have to start thinking about running a marathon or doing 100 push-ups (but who knows, you might find that appealing later on - don't underestimate the motivating power of starting a workout routine).

When we think of exercise, we think of gym sessions, lycra, exercise classes. I never found these appealing, because I felt too self-conscious. I have good news for you if you feel the same: you don't need a gym or a class to get fit. You can do it from home. You don't even need any special equipment to begin with. The only thing you will need is some comfortable clothing, and the determination to stick to your new healthy regime.

Start with Movement

Or rather, start by taking an honest look at how much movement there is in your day. When do you exercise? How many steps do you take? Write down your daily activity levels and use this as a benchmark from which to build on.

Technology has meant that a very large majority of us work from offices; we move very little. You might spend 8-10 hours a day at a desk, then another 1-2 hours sat on a train or bus, and perhaps 3-4 hours in front of the television at night. That means an average day is made up of short transitions from one seat to another. This lack of exercise is one of the reasons for weight gain. Changing this is vital to reach a healthy weight and rebalance hormones.

Before you start thinking about getting an elliptical machine for the office, work out if you can make any small changes to increase the level of movement in your daily life. My suggestion is that you begin by monitoring and increasing your daily step count. Yes, it can be as simple as going out for a nice long walk.

In Chapter 9, I'll share tips to help you create a new morning routine that supports healthy habits. You could incorporate a walk before you officially begin your day. The thought of waking up and crushing a gym session might not be your cup of tea, and honestly, I don't blame you! When I was not feeling my best, there is no way I wanted to be struggling my way through a workout in front of other people, especially when my fitness levels were lower than that of your average gym-goer. Add to that the stress of waiting for a treadmill to be free, and having to wipe other people's sweat off equipment, this is not a very zen start to the day. But a walk, on the other hand, is a great way to improve your fitness levels in a gentle, stress-free way.

Getting up and going out for a walk in the morning is a great way to get rid of PCOS symptoms. Any cardiovascular activity helps reduce insulin resistance, and if you combine regular cardio with resistance training (more on that in a second), you will see a noticeable difference in the weight that you carry around your mid-region.

If walking in the morning isn't your thing, no problem. Try a lunchtime walk instead, or a walk after dinner. You can also incorporate mindfulness and meditation in your walking routine, perfect for letting go of the stress of the day, or setting intention for the day ahead. If you can walk in nature, even better!

There is a bonus reason for exercising, and that is mood. Exercising boosts your levels of serotonin, our very own feel-good neurotransmitter. The better you feel, the easier it is to stick to a new routine, and the better able you are to deal with stress. Both of these aspects are very helpful when it comes to healing PCOS.

Here are a few ways to include more movement into your day and begin experiencing the benefits for yourself:

- Take the stairs, or walk up escalators.
- Get off the train or bus one stop earlier, or park your car a little further away, and walk the rest of the way.
- Go for a brisk walk at lunchtime.
- Get your family involved - get out in nature at the weekend.
- Reach out to friends or colleagues and organize regular group walks.
- Use TV time for good, by doing stretches, jumping jacks, squats or half press-ups during the advert breaks.

When I was working full time and trying to implement some cardio into my life, I suggested to a colleague that we go out for a walk at lunch instead of sitting in our usual place every day. It became a very enjoyable activity. My energy levels improved and I felt less workplace stress. Walking has benefits for the mind as well as the body, and that is a good rule of thumb when choosing exercises for PCOS. Try to find activities that you can do mindfully and ones that allow you to engage with your inner health.

Strength Training and Core Exercises

In order to maximize the benefits of the gentle cardio, it's a good idea to combine it with strength and core exercises.

Strength training is particularly helpful for changing your body composition and building muscle, which is a great way to increase your metabolism (how many calories you burn at rest) and therefore lose weight.

Building resistance into your workouts can be as easy as finding some water. Swimming and water aerobics are a fantastic way to burn fat and pump up your heart rate. The resistance of your body going through the water is enough to give your body an all-over workout. What's more, it is low impact, so no risk of injuries. Swimming is another great exercise to do mindfully. You can let the water lift you up and wash away any stress or tension you feel.

Another type of exercise that works particularly well with PCOS sufferers is HIIT, or High-Intensity Interval Training. This is more intense than a brisk walk, as the name itself would suggest, but where cardio is great for overall health and mood, HIIT can actually work wonders for slimming down your waist and burning fat.

HIIT is basically bursts of intensive aerobic exercise, performed with short breaks - one example is a spin class. If it feels a bit too overwhelming to be doing this on your own, get a group of girls together to try out a class or make it a social event. Just one class like this a week will have a big impact on your weight loss. You can also try HIIT at home - there are plenty of workout apps that guide you through short workouts you can do in as little as 10 minutes (such as the 7M app). These are great if you're pressed for time but still want to get your heart rate up and your muscles working.

Get Outside

Going outdoors can also take the headache out of exercise and make it feel less like a chore. When kids are running about and playing, they are not thinking about how many calories they are losing or how many steps they are adding to their Fitbit. They are just concentrating on how much fun they are having. Try to build more outdoor activity like that into your week. Research what's around you - most places will have a park or gardens where you can wander. Alternatively, see if there are any tennis courts or outdoor tracks nearby.

Yoga and Pilates

Yoga and Pilates actually deserve a special mention when it comes to great exercises for PCOS.

Yoga is a 5000-year-old practice, originally developed to improve health on all levels: physical, mental and spiritual. The word yoga means "to yoke" or "concentration," it promotes a calmer state of mind while strengthening and stretching your muscles and improving balance. There are many types of yoga available, from the restorative yin yoga, where poses are held for a long time, to the energizing Bikram yoga done in studios heated between 90-108 degrees Fahrenheit.

Pilates was developed as a healing strategy for injured dancers, and combines core strength (abdomen, obliques, lower back, glutes and thighs) with flexibility, endurance, coordination and balance, making it a great all-round workout for your body.

Both of these practices have an undercurrent of mindfulness and meditation that are helpful to beat stress and improve your overall mood. As a result, regularly practicing yoga and Pilates can have more far-reaching effects than just a post-exercise glow. Practices like yoga traveled to the West in the '60s and '70s as part of the hippie movement, which also birthed a lot of the Western meditation and spiritual movement. It's no wonder that with our ever-increasing workloads and the growing stress of modern life, the thought of tapping into some Eastern healing practices for an hour a week is extremely appealing.

Practicing mindful exercises will help to improve your awareness of the link between your physical health and your mindset, which is vital to your healing and recovery process as well as creating an environment that will improve fertility levels.

The examples in this section are intended as a guide to help you on your way. The most important thing is to find an exercise that you enjoy, because if you enjoy what you're doing, you will find it easy to stick to. There is no right or wrong way, what matters is that you are moving your body. That could take different forms, so try not to restrict yourself. Putting on your favorite song and dancing in your kitchen is as good a form of exercise as any, perhaps even more so if it puts a smile on your face.

CHAPTER NINE:

QUALITY SLEEP IS THE KEY - YOUR NEW NIGHT-TIME & MORNING ROUTINES

Small changes all add up to a big difference. Overhauling your diet, increasing the amount of movement in your day, and practicing some form of meditation - these are all going to have a positive impact on your health and your PCOS symptoms. But we often forget one vital thing: sleep.

While no studies link sleep problems directly with PCOS, it's easy to see how poor sleep can impact both physical and mental health. After all, we know how irritable we can be if we haven't had enough sleep. That extra stress only makes it more likely that we will turn to comfort foods, or stimulants. And few people feel motivated to exercise when they wake up exhausted. More stress equals higher levels of cortisol, equals more inflammation, which can worsen PCOS symptoms. Clearly, even without a direct link, sleep is an important part of your healing process.

As I've mentioned a few times, healing PCOS requires a holistic approach. Simply eating fewer cheeseburgers, walking more, or sleeping longer may not on their own take away your PCOS symptoms, but when you combine them all, you will notice a marked difference.

You will also find that following the advice in other chapters on eating healthily and working out will affect how tired you are. It is often the case that we sleep poorly because our bodies are too sedentary. If you sit at a desk all day followed by sitting on a couch all night, then it is not surprising that your body is not switching over to sleep mode at the given time. The body is a well-tuned athletic machine. If you are not using some of that natural energy, then you might find that you experience an ongoing feeling of lethargy rather than the natural rhythm of sleep and wake cycles.

The Impact of Sleep

Consider the impact that a bad night's sleep has on your overall day. We have all been there, and probably more recently than we would like to remember! Whether it is that we are not getting enough hours of sleep, that we are waking up at regular intervals, or that we are sleeping in an uncomfortable position, not sleeping well is enough to produce noticeable effects throughout our day. From bags under the eyes to brain fog, increased cravings to increased irritability, we have all experienced the effects of not getting quality sleep.

Thankfully, these issues can often be resolved by an early night and a deposit of some extra sleep hours into the proverbial sleep bank. Within 24 hours, we are usually back to normal. But what if your sleep is disrupted every night? This situation is more common than you would think. Due to the way sleep happens, it might not be as simple as just getting an extra few hours a night.

Sleep can be broken up into four stages:

1. **Falling asleep stage**: Your eyes are closed, but you haven't yet fallen asleep.
2. **Light sleep stage**: Your heart rate slows and your body is getting ready for deep sleep. You can easily be woken up at this stage.
3. **Deep sleep stage**: You are in a deeper state of rest. It would be harder to wake you up at this stage.
4. **Rapid eye movement (REM) stage**: You dream; your glymphatic system (the brain's detox mechanism) is activated.

The first three stages are known as non-REM stages, and usually last up to 15 minutes each. Stages 2, 3 and 4 are repeated throughout the night. The first REM stage usually happens 90 minutes after you fall asleep and lasts around 10 minutes. You then go back through stages 2, 3 and 4, with each REM stage getting longer as the night goes on. The longer you can be in REM sleep, the better for your health.

But many of us fail to get uninterrupted, quality sleep. We struggle to fall asleep, or wake up during the night.

One of the reasons why this happens (and the easiest one to fix), is because we are completely disconnected from natural light and dark cycles. We have special cells in our eyes that communicate with the brain depending on your environment. If you are around short-wavelength light (such as street lights, blue light from phones and televisions, or the light that comes from a clear blue sky), these cells tell your brain to make hormones like cortisol and ghrelin - hormones that wake us up and make us feel hungry (why is why you may feel very awake and kind of hungry after you watch a late-night program). As the day gets dark, they tell your brain to produce melatonin, that makes you drowsy and gets the body ready for sleep. But dusk doesn't mean darkness any more, and this excess of light in the evening makes it harder to fall asleep and harder to stay asleep.

In order to reset your sleep cycle and get plenty of time in REM sleep, you have to create the right conditions, and this might mean you have to change your night-time routine. Here are my tips to get your started.

- **Set the scene**: Make your bedroom a haven for sleep. Get rid of televisions and computers, invest in some black-out curtains or an eye mask, and make sure your bed is comfortable and the right temperature for you. Pick colors that you find calming.
- **No more blue light**: Change the lightbulbs in your home to warmer, yellow lights. You can download an app that changes your phone and tablet screen light from blue to red in the evenings (you can also switch

your phone or tablet to "nighttime mode"). Remember that as part of your digital detox, you are not checking your phone for 1-2 hours before going to bed.

- **Avoid stressful activities before sleep**: The evening news or cliff-hanger series will raise your stress and your cortisol levels. Watch them earlier in the day and keep the evening free for more relaxing activities, like reading or getting creative.
- **Use essential oils**: Lavender and blue chamomile are beautiful scents that will carry you into a restful sleep. Use them in an oil diffuser, or take a warm bath with relaxing oil blends before bed.
- **Limit stimulants**: If you're a fan of fizzy or caffeinated drinks, avoid them from mid-afternoon. Swap your coffee for decaf or herbal tea from around 2pm.

Your New Morning Routine

Just like changing your evenings transforms your sleep, changing your morning will transform your day. It's true. That first hour after you wake up holds the key to either a great day, or a bad day.

Morning routines can be difficult to change, mostly because we have got into bad habits and can't see how to do things differently. Difficult, but certainly not impossible. And it can even be easy once you experience how much better you feel just by shifting your morning routine a little.

Ideally, you want to be able to give yourself 30 to 60 minutes before you have to get ready for work. This might mean you need to get up a little earlier, but saving time by not checking your phone first thing in the morning (remember, digital detox!) will help with that. What this extra time enables you to connect with yourself, set your intention for the day, and provide you with some you time - something that is severely lacking in our increasingly busy lives.

Right now you might be thinking - why do I need to change my morning routine? And the answer is simply: if you don't change the basics, nothing can change. Look at these two scenarios.

Your alarm goes off, you hit snooze three times before you finally drag yourself out of bed - you feel exhausted after a poor night's sleep. You stomp around the house, stubbing your toe on the coffee-table as you do so. You brew a strong coffee and sip it quickly while scrolling through Instagram, before leaving the house in a hurry, grabbing a pastry, not getting a seat on the train, and getting to work in a foul mood.

Your alarm goes off and you wake feeling refreshed after a restful sleep. You get up, drink a glass of water and do a ten-minute workout. You then sit quietly for a five to ten minutes guided meditation. You make yourself a cup of tea and eat the healthy breakfast you prepared the night before, spend ten to fifteen minutes journaling (either writing a gratitude list, or setting your intention for the day, or exploring how you feel in that moment). You leave the house on time, check your social media on the train, and arrive at work feeling ready to take on the day.

It is obvious which of the two mornings results in lower levels of stress and higher levels of happiness.

In just half an hour, you can exercise, meditate, and organize your day, thereby giving yourself the best start. We've talked about exercise in Chapter 8. So now, I want you to take a piece of paper and design your very own positive morning routine. What does it look like? What time do you need to get up to give yourself enough time to do everything serenely? How do you want to feel as you practice this? Once you have created this new morning routine, put it into practice. You will be amazed and delighted how much of a difference this makes to your mood and overall health.

Supplements and Sleep Aids

Some supplements and accessories can assist you in a comfortable sleep. Melatonin is a naturally occurring hormone in our bodies that is closely tied to sleep. Our levels of melatonin rise at night and lower in the morning, helping to regulate our sleep and wake cycles. Melatonin can be taken as a supplement, and can be effective at helping you achieve a restful night's sleep.

Other aids can stimulate the melatonin production in your system by replicating the natural conditions of day and night, to encourage waking at the appropriate time. Some alarm clocks mimic the rise of dawn light to wake you. If you travel a lot, you can purchase a device known as the Human Charger which works through your headphones and reduces the effects of jet lag by rectifying your natural sleep cycle as quickly as possible.

You can try sleep monitors, like the WHOOP strap, to track your sleep. Free sleep apps are also available. However, since you'll want to keep screens to a minimum, I don't tend to recommend these. Give yourself a chance to rebalance your sleep by putting the strategies in this chapter into practice first - most people find that's all they need.

Remember that reducing stress levels is key to helping your hormones rebalance and ridding yourself of PCOS symptoms. Starting your day in a positive way - with healthy habits and through loving self-care - and ensuring you get proper sleep, will support the health of both body and mind, and help you banish PCOS symptoms for good.

CHAPTER TEN:
SOME EXTRA TIPS AND ADVICE

I've outlined the main areas of PCOS - its causes, risk factors, and what you can do to rebalance your hormones. You are not alone - many of the symptoms you experience are also experienced by other women with PCOS. The remedies and strategies for reducing the symptoms work for most women. There is a danger of information overload. Honestly, if you search diligently enough on the internet, you will find a contrary argument to just about every health tip out there, so understandably, it can be hard to know where to turn and what information to trust.

For that reason, I thought I would use this chapter to share some additional strategies to top off your PCOS wellness journey. This book is intended to be a reference guide for you to come back to, so if you find some information here that you do not think you can realistically implement into your life right now, try revisiting the chapter and reconsidering it after you have achieved the other key changes, particularly in the areas of diet, fitness, and sleep.

Plastic Bottles

We have already briefly mentioned this, but it's worth revising quickly. It's a topic that some people dismiss as a conspiracy theory: the impact of plastic bottles on PCOS symptoms. More and more, we are learning about the detrimental effect plastic has on our lives. Plastic does not degrade, it remains in the environment for thousands of years. When you consider that the majority of plastics are single use - in other words, they serve a very short-term purpose, for example wrapping a broccoli, or the plastic lining in a take-away cup - you get an idea of how nonsensical our society is. We are polluting the planet - there are plastic islands in the Pacific Ocean that are larger than France. And we are polluting ourselves. One particular compound in plastic, Bisphenol A, commonly referred to as BPA, can exacerbate PCOS symptoms. A recent study conducted at the University of Athens found that not only were BPA levels significantly higher in women with PCOS (30-40% higher), but that increased exposure to BPA could potentially cause PCOS. As BPA accumulates in the body, it increases the level of androgens in the system, which, as we know, is a key factor in PCOS.

The first thing to do to minimize exposure is to stop using plastic drinking bottles entirely. Always drink from a stainless steel or glass water bottles or ceramic mugs, and always store food in ceramic, metal, or glass containers. If you absolutely cannot avoid plastic bottles in some circumstances, then don't leave them out in the sun and always discard them immediately after use. Also, avoid using plastic for any type of cooking, particularly microwaving, and remember that even regular dishwasher use can degrade the plastic in your containers and storage tubs enough to make them dangerous.

Herbs, Spices, and Supplements

Your best chance of tackling PCOS is to eat a balanced diet and engage in regular exercise. A balanced diet is one that includes plenty of whole foods, but also plenty of herbs and spices. In Chapter 7, we looked at the importance of antioxidants. Herbs and spices deliver these in abundance through their volatile oils and plant pigments. Whether it is oregano, rosemary, mint, cumin, black pepper, garlic, cilantro, parsley, paprika, turmeric, tarragon, fennel seeds, etc. The list is endless, and they add both flavor and a health boost to your meals.

While no single food will deliver healing on its own, some supplements can really help to manage your symptoms. They are not magic pills, however, and will only deliver benefits if taken alongside healthy lifestyle changes.

Magnesium and iron are two minerals that occur naturally in the body, but in PCOS sufferers, they may be present in lower quantities than is required for optimal health. You can increase your magnesium and iron intake by eating foods that are rich in these minerals - almonds, cashews, and bananas for magnesium, and spinach and broccoli for iron. Most good quality multivitamins will contain both these minerals.

Women need 18-27 mg of iron per day and 310-360 mg of magnesium per day.

Here is a list of my favorite PCOS-symptom-busting supplements. I strongly recommend working with either a holistic endocrine specialist or herbalist who will be able to advise which of these supplements will work best for you, based on your needs and current health status:

- Chromium - helps to balance blood sugar and improve insulin sensitivity. Recommended intake for women is 25-45 micrograms per day.
- Cinnamon - also helps balance blood sugar levels. Delicious added to oats, sprinkled over apples, or added to coffee.
- Turmeric - a powerful anti-inflammatory and antioxidant that will help to reduce inflammation and relieve menstrual pain. Add to smoothies, curries and dressings, or make a coconut turmeric latte.
- Ashwagandha - an adaptogen, which means it helps your body to deal with stress and can help alleviate depression. Best taken in capsule form (the taste is very bitter). Suggested dosage between 500 and 1000 milligrams per day.
- Black Cohosh (cimicifuga racemosa) - boosts fertility, improves the balance of luteinizing hormone and follicle stimulating hormone. Can help reduce PMS symptoms. Suggested dosage between 20-40 mg per day.
- Licorice (glycyrrhiza glabra) - Helps reduce androgen

hormones while improving ovulation rates. Suggested dosage 3.5 grams licorice containing 7% glycyrrhizic acid) per day for 2 months.

Intermittent Fasting

One way of eating has been studied in relation to its impact on insulin sensitivity: intermittent fasting (IF). You can incorporate intermittent fasting into your life quite easily - let me show you how.

When people think of fasting, they think of eating nothing for days at a time. That is one type of fasting, but it's not the kind I'm advocating here. You can intermittently fast simply by changing when you eat breakfast and dinner.

Intermittent fasting can be your secret weapon when it comes to beating PCOS. It reduces inflammation and helps you lose weight. In an animal study published in the journal Nutrition, scientists gave two groups of mice either a high fat or a high fructose diet for 8 weeks. Half of these mice were then put though an intermittent fasting routine for 4 weeks - without changing their diet. Interestingly, despite carrying on with pro-inflammatory diets, the mice that ate intermittently had fewer inflammatory markers than mice that ate normally. Conclusion: intermittent fasting reduces inflammation and can therefore help you overcome PCOS.

If it can do that without dietary change, imagine how beneficial it can be combined with a healthier diet and exercise

How does intermittent fasting work? It comes down to giving your body some time out of the "fed" state. For 3 to 5 hours after you eat, your body is busy digesting food, breaking it down, absorbing it, eliminating it... that's one of the reasons many people feel sleepy after a meal.

These days, we are encouraged to eat every 3 to 4 hours, which means we're always either eating or digesting. With intermittent fasting, you can give your body time in the "fasted" state - this happens around 8 to 12 hours after you eat. At this time, your body is no longer busy digesting, and it can get on with rejuvenating, detoxing and healing.

There's no single way to intermittently fast. Some people do 20/4 - which is when you eat within a 4-hour period but fast the rest of the time. This is known as the Warrior Diet, and, though it is effective, it is perhaps too hardcore if you are new to intermittent fasting. Remember that stress is part of PCOS and we want to keep stress to a minimum.

Another way is to try 16/8, which is much easier to incorporate into your day. Here, you eat in an 8-hour window, for example between 10am and 6pm, or between 12pm and 8pm, or whatever time-frame suits you, and fast the rest of the time. This means you can have tea or herbal tea, black coffee, and water the rest of the time. You can make water a bit more interesting by infusing it with fresh ginger, turmeric, mint, lemon, lime. Since intermittent fasting also helps your body to detox, it's a good idea to drink plenty of water to help your body flush out those toxins.

If you want to ease into intermittent fasting, a great place to start is simply to give your body at least 12 hours between dinner and breakfast the next day. So, if you usually have dinner at 7pm, delay your breakfast till after 7am.

I've found intermittent fasting to be incredibly helpful. It gave me more energy during the day, and saved me a lot of time in the mornings. My preferred window of eating is between 11am and 7pm, which meant I didn't need to make breakfast. After a couple of days, I no longer felt hungry at that time anyway, because intermittent fasting helps balance blood sugar and therefore normalizes appetite and cravings.

Acupressure

Another very interesting area for PCOS sufferers is acupressure. Similar to acupuncture, the process of applying pressure on certain points on the body, particularly hands and feet, to stimulate the body's internal healing system and target problem areas. Issues like bloating, headaches, and menstrual cramps can be relieved with acupressure techniques, and some claim there are fertility benefits when acupressure is used in conjunction with a holistic health approach. While you shouldn't get acupressure if you are pregnant or have a heart condition, it is otherwise a perfectly safe and non-invasive procedure that could potentially alleviate some of your symptoms. There is no harm in giving it a try. Keep a note of how you feel in the days before and after the treatment in your journal so that you can track whether it is contributing to your healing process.

There are three points on your foot that correlate to key areas of the body affected by PCOS. By learning where these pressure points are, you can practice acupressure on your own! Your feet are full of nerve endings and touchpoints that relate to different areas of your body. That's why a foot massage can feel so refreshing and relaxing. It is, in essence, a whole-body massage as well.

Three areas in particular that we want to tackle for PCOS symptoms would be our ovaries, uterus, and the lymphatic drainage system, which alleviates bloating and the symptoms of menstrual cramps. For your ovaries, you want to apply pressure approximately one thumb width below the ankle bone on the outside of your foot, pressing down with your thumb as if you are pulling back towards your heel. For your uterus, you want to apply the same technique in the same area, but this time work on the inside of your foot. Treat these areas separately and massage each one for around 1 minute, twice per day on each foot for maximum results.

To support your lymphatic system, move the pressure to the top of your foot, just below the space between your first and second toe. Again, pull back towards you as you massage, and do this for around a minute twice a day on each foot. If you are prone to pain in your breasts just before your period, the lymphatic acupressure method could work wonders.

#PCOS on Instagram

The modern way to self-diagnose is increasingly done on the internet, and there is a growing number of health experts who share their knowledge and insights on social media. As I have mentioned previously, I first became aware of Chiara Ferragni's story through Instagram, and at the time, I found it almost by accident. The joy and hope I felt reading her story was life-changing. I feel so grateful every time someone of that stature uses her platform to help other women by sharing her story. The replies to her post were also very inspiring, full of other women's stories about getting pregnant with PCOS, and lovely comments in support of women who were going through PCOS-related fertility struggles.

By searching the hashtag #PCOS regularly, I found success stories, exercise tips, help with my diet, and a growing number of experts and fellow PCOS sufferers who were actually sharing insightful and refreshing advice. I know I have spent at least two chapters now telling you to put your phone away for a large percentage of the day, but when you do have it back in your hand, do some research and spend some time looking through these organic online communities. It goes without saying that you should be wary of anyone offering miracle cures - no single supplement or treatment will magically heal PCOS. It's a journey.

I hope the online PCOS community brings you the same level of support that it brought me. I might even see you there!

FINAL WORDS

I can't thank you enough for taking the time to read this book and allowing me to be a small part of your PCOS journey. When I first got diagnosed, I never would have thought I would end up writing a book to help change the lives of other women with this condition. It has been a dream come true. It just goes to show that PCOS is not a life sentence, and that light can shine through the darkness.

It is so important to spread the message of wellness and to share our stories of weight loss, mood management, wellbeing, and even pregnancy! I have been blessed with welcoming a son into the world naturally, even though at one point, we thought it would be impossible. I credit that to the lifestyle changes I made - changes you can make too. It also helped me to read the stories of other women who were just like me and managed to become pregnant after a PCOS diagnosis. It filled me with so much hope and created a mild obsession with learning about how wellbeing, lifestyle, fitness, and good daily habits contribute to improved health.

Overhauling your diet and changing your lifestyle has far-reaching effects in your external life, and it can also radically transform your internal life. From digestive problems to extreme anxiety, I have experienced just how much of my life can be transformed by simply changing the foods I eat and the activities I do.

I started this journey, like you, with some apprehension and fear at the idea of transforming my life so drastically. But after putting into practice the suggestions in this book, I've never looked back. So don't be afraid. Just take that first step. A wellness-based approach to PCOS is gathering momentum, and real support for this movement is growing, even within the medical profession. The female body is a delicately balanced but highly resilient model, and I hope after reading this book, you will start to realize just what your body is capable of. I hope you see that it is possible for you also to see transformational change in your life.

We have covered the basics of PCOS, and looked at how you can improve your wellbeing from several angles - diet, fitness, and mindset. Every journey starts with a single step, and every morning you can decide to show yourself love and help your body to heal.

The reason I covered more than just diet and exercise was that when I attempted dieting and exercising without focusing on my state of mind, I ended up not sticking to good habits. I would start to see results, but then I would be so moody or tired that I would resort to sugar and caffeine. It wasn't until I really took the time to understand my moods and tackle my depression, that I was able to make the changes stick. This is where your belief in yourself comes in. Believe that you can heal. Your body knows what to do, it simply needs the tools to do it - healthy food, daily movement, and loving thoughts.

That is the most important step - believe in yourself.

I am grateful that I had an extremely understanding partner, particularly in the early days when I was trying to get a handle on my emotions and control my mindset. There were good days and bad days, but I was always reassured and encouraged by the wonderful and supportive women that I met along the way.

My wish when writing this book was to convey all that I learned. I hope I have provided you with a strong and solid foundation with which to recover from PCOS. I wish you the best of luck with your journey and encourage you to share your own story online or in person.

Every woman can benefit from more information on wellness. I want to shout from the rooftops about the benefits of a holistic approach to health, and I would ask you to please join me in sharing that message far and wide.

I know you can do it. I know you have the willpower and the stamina to make these changes and make over your life, and that you can serve as an inspiration to other women to do the same.

I wish you all the success in the world with your transformation.

You can do this.

Maggie

Printed in Great Britain
by Amazon